Comments on **Taking Control of Cancer** *from readers*

"A very useful and immensely supportive book, both for individuals cing cancer and for their loved ones . . ."

Dr Jo Clough, Senior Lecturer and cancer survivor,
University of Southampton

'I think this book will be extremely useful to anyone recently facing a cancer diagnosis. Things have improved beyond all recognition in the seven years since my husband was diagnosed . . . So this book will be a fantastic starting point for anyone facing the long uncertain road of cancer treatment."

Caroline Wallis, Hampshire

'The book itself is clear, concise and well written, but it is the patients' experiences that are the most compelling aspect. It is exceptionally difficult for anyone like me on the other side of the coin, to understand he feelings and fears that patients confront on a day-to-day basis. But his book, and the shared experiences within it, have helped me to cope nd, more importantly, helped my father. A fascinating read."

Emily Hicks, London

Taking Control of Cancer

Everything you want to know about cancer – getting information, treatment options, choices, self-help

Beverley van der Molen

Patient Information Officer, Royal Marsden NHS Trust

CLASS PUBLISHING · LONDON

© Beverley van der Molen 2003
© Class Publishing (London) Ltd

Printing history
First published 2003

The author and the publishers welcome feedback from the users of this book. Please contact the publishers.

**Class Publishing (London) Ltd, Barb House, Barb Mews,
London W6 7PA
Telephone: 020 7371 2119
Fax: 020 7371 2878 [International +4420]
Website: www.class.co.uk**

The information presented in this book is accurate and current to the best of the authors' knowledge. The author and publisher, however, make no guarantee as to, and assume no responsibility for, the correctness, sufficiency or completeness of such information or recommendation. The reader is advised to consult a doctor regarding all aspects of individual health care.

A CIP catalogue record for this book is available from the British Library

ISBN 1 85959 091 8

Edited by Richenda Milton-Thompson

Indexed by Valerie Elliston

Typeset by Martin Bristow

Printed and bound in Finland by WS Bookwell, Juva

Contents

Acknowledgements

Communication involves the exchange of thoughts, feelings or ideas. Just as communication cannot happen in isolation, this book would not have been written without the encouragement and contributions of the many people from whose experiences I have drawn.

Therefore, my special thanks go to the members and users of the Cancer Resource Centre who have contributed in so many ways. In addition to the many conversations about what they have seen as important communication issues, they have also provided accounts of their experiences. It takes courage to reflect back on an experience as challenging as living with cancer, to relive the many different emotions that are inevitably generated.

I would also like to thank Petra Griffiths, the Director of the Cancer Resource Centre, for her constant support throughout and Stephanie Jacobs who provided much of the inspiration for this book. Their experience and understanding of cancer, and of communication has been invaluable.

In order to preserve the confidentiality of people whose stories are recounted in the book, names and other identifying details have been changed.

Finally, I would like to thank my husband, Rick, for his patience and understanding while writing this book.

Beverley van der Molen

Foreword

Hearing that you have cancer is an overwhelming experience. Often the shock means that you can't remember what was said when the diagnosis was delivered. This is an important book for people with cancer and their carers. Having so much information in one place will clear up confusion. People will be able to come back to topics raised in the hospital setting when they seem relevant. Diagnosis and treatment are covered as well as longer term information and support, which becomes significant when people are no longer having regular treatment, and start to feel isolated. An important aspect of this book is the way it goes on to explain how you can exert an influence on the future of cancer services, so that no experience need be wasted.

Many individuals with cancer have contributed to this book by reflecting on their experience and how they have changed as a result. These personal accounts are very honest in their assessment of the impact of cancer, and I found a number of the stories of how people have responded to the challenges that cancer brings both inspiring and moving.

Much of my own cancer experience at UCLH was excellent. My wish is for everyone diagnosed with cancer today to have access to good communication, the recognition of the need for choice, and the tangible atmosphere of excellence. This book brings this vision closer by giving people tools to enable them to ask directly for what they need.

Petra Griffiths

Petra Griffiths
Director, The Cancer Resource Centre

Introduction

Cancer is such an emotive word, raising all kinds of feelings and questions. And it is because of the emotional dimension that communication can be so difficult.

No one knows how they will react to a diagnosis of cancer until they are confronted with it. Nor do they know what they will need in terms of information, support, or even treatment until some time after being given that diagnosis.

This book covers the emotional and information needs of people who have been diagnosed with cancer, and those involved with them. It aims to diminish some of the fears surrounding cancer that make communication difficult and, as a result, to help you feel more comfortable when talking about cancer as you realise that what you feel is not unique to you.

Access to information about cancer, and reading other peoples' stories, will make it clear to readers that cancer is not necessarily a death sentence. This is particularly true in the short term. Indeed, many people continue to enjoy a good quality of life for years after being diagnosed as having cancer, some eventually dying from other causes entirely.

Good communication lays the foundation for a good relationship with your health care team, which will help you to be treated as an individual and to be supported throughout your cancer experience. However, it is not only communicating effectively with health professionals that is important. Good communication can make the world of difference when talking to your family, friends and work colleagues and, if you are a parent, to your children. Misunderstandings can arise in all these areas when there are communication difficulties. Communication is very much a two-way process and is based on a shared understanding and language.

There is no right or wrong way of coping with living with cancer. It is very individual and you will probably find that the way you deal with the situation will change constantly. You may well feel that your world has turned upside down and is spiralling out of control. The world of medicine can seem very alien when you first hear unfamiliar medical terminology and meet many different health professionals. This is bound to have an effect on how you cope.

1

Information can play an important part in helping people understand more about their illness and provide them with options for managing the situation. When you understand what is happening to you, you are likely to feel more in control of your life. Information can help you cope with both the practical aspects of the illness and its treatments, and manage any fear and anxiety you may feel.

How do doctors deal with the emotions of their patients when informing them they have cancer and at the same time deal with their own feelings? How do doctors know whether their patients want complete honesty or if they only want to hear information that is positive? How do individuals ensure that they are given appropriate information and support? What can they do if something goes wrong? How can they ensure that their voices are heard? There are no clear-cut answers to help people manage, but greater insight will inevitably lead to greater understanding that can only benefit everyone.

How individuals cope with cancer depends on many factors including previous experiences and social support networks. The personal stories of people living with cancer can highlight instances of communication working well, and not so well. We can learn from other people's experiences where the potential areas of difficulty might be, and absorb practical suggestions about how we too can communicate effectively with health professionals and others, in order to get the information we need.

What is cancer?

The term 'cancer' actually refers to a group of diseases, but what they all have in common is that they attack the cells, tiny particles invisible to the naked eye but essentially the 'building blocks' that make up every part of our body. As the whole body, including the blood, is made up of these building blocks, cancers can occur anywhere in the body.

A normal cell will divide periodically. In a young person this process is frequent in order to allow for growth, but it continues to be necessary in adulthood as the cells must replace themselves in order to maintain body tissues in good repair. Sometimes this process goes wrong, however, and the cells start to divide in an uncontrolled manner resulting in a swelling or tumour. These swellings can be either 'benign' or 'malignant'.

Benign tumours can usually be removed by surgery and are unlikely to cause further problems. Malignant, or cancerous, growths however can spread to other organs throughout the body. If a small clump of cancerous cells from a tumour in one part of your body settles somewhere else, cancer will then develop in this new place too. Because cancer cells can spread to organs such as the lungs or liver – which are necessary for life – untreated cancer anywhere in the body can be life-threatening.

Which cancers are you most likely to encounter?

Some cancers occur more often than others, though this also tends to vary from one country to another. Every year 200,000 people are diagnosed with cancer in England. There are over 200 different types of cancer, although the four major types, lung, breast, prostate and colorectal, account for over half of all cases diagnosed.

◆ Breast cancer is the most common cancer in women, accounting for nearly 30 per cent of all new female cancers. In men there are around 300 cases each year.

◆ Lung cancer is the most common cancer in men and the third most common in women.

◆ Prostate is currently the second most common cancer in men after lung cancer. However, while the number of people developing lung cancer is decreasing, the number of men developing prostate cancer is increasing.

◆ Colorectal or bowel cancer is the third most commonly diagnosed cancer in the UK. It is more likely to occur in older people.

You can find out more statistics about cancer on Cancer Research UK's website (see page 154).

How to use this book

You may not want to read the whole of this book at one time, so each chapter has been designed in order to be read on its own. This means you will find some of the issues discussed will be covered in more than one chapter. The following chapters bring together the different stages of living with cancer, highlighting the various emotions and questions where good communication can make a difference.

Uncertainty and diagnosis – lets you know that the shock, confusion and anger you may experience in the period surrounding a diagnosis of cancer are perfectly normal. This is not to deny they are unpleasant, but you can be reassured that you will regain some sense of control, even if you will never again enjoy perfect health. Countless others have been through this particular rite of passage and have come out the other side. So will you.

An introduction to cancer services – outlines what can be expected from the beginning of your 'cancer experience' and focuses on current cancer services. It gives a foundation on which to build blocks of information that will help you to understand and live with cancer.

Communicating with health professionals – discusses the various reactions that individuals may experience when hearing information that changes their view of their future for the worse. It also looks at some of the barriers to good communication and ways of overcoming these barriers.

Sharing the diagnosis – acknowledges that cancer also affects families, partners, friends and work colleagues. This chapter goes on to explore some of the ways in which information can be shared with them.

Treatment options – discusses the information you need to help you understand about the different treatments available, so you can take part in making decisions about your own treatment and care.

Coping with cancer – looks at the impact that cancer has on family, friends and work, and the different kinds of support that are available. This chapter also discusses moving on when treatment has finished.

What can you do to help yourself? – looks at different ways of accessing support, also at the potential of complementary therapies.

Other barriers to communication – explores some of the issues that may create further communication difficulties such as sight, hearing and language difficulties, as well as cultural differences, and approaches to overcoming them. Cancer may also affect identity and self-image, further barriers to communication.

Being heard – looks at what you can do if you are unhappy with any aspect of your care, such as getting a second opinion or making a complaint. This chapter also discusses how you can use your experience to benefit others, both in the present and in the future.

Seeking information – brings together many information resources on the different areas covered in this book, and gives advice on how to use them.

You will find the stories of different people interwoven with the text. These are real people who are, or who have been patients, although their names have been changed. They have trodden this road before you, have experienced the rage, bewilderment and fear that accompanies diagnosis and early treatment, and have come to terms with living with cancer. While your experience will be unique to you, they share their experiences with you in the hope that you may feel less alone.

1
Uncertainty and diagnosis

Few people will go through life without being touched by cancer in some way, whether personally, or through family, friends or colleagues. Our own experiences and what we read and hear through the media influence our understanding of cancer.

One of the biggest problems with any new experience is recognising what it is that you need to know. It is difficult to think about what information will be helpful when you are still coming to terms with your diagnosis. So how can you be sure you know what questions to ask? Your doctors will recommend treatment on the basis of research findings and their own experience of treating your kind of cancer. They will also take into account the stage your cancer is at, your general health and your own wishes.

People respond to a cancer diagnosis in many different ways.

My experience began in 1997. Now I remember that very clearly because it was the day of the general election. I'd reached my 50th birthday and was called for a mammogram [screening for breast cancer]. *I had the test and thought that was it because I'd had many mammograms before that. Then I had this letter saying that they would like me to come and have a second one but there was nothing to worry about. So when I went back for the second one, they did a needle aspiration and said they'd let me know the following Monday. Well two weeks went by and I heard nothing and I thought 'Oh well, it will be OK then.' I went to my GP to find out if they'd had the result, thinking 'If two weeks have gone by and they haven't informed me, it must be good news because if it wasn't they would let me know.' To stop me worrying, my GP said he'd ask his secretary to get them to fax the result through. I remember sitting there, I remember hearing the word 'carcinoma' and I knew what that meant. I don't remember anything else. I remember walking out of the surgery going round the corner, voting and walking home. I got home, sat in the chair and I couldn't move. It was the strangest thing. And I sat and I sat and I couldn't move. It was just like me watching somebody else. It was me doing it but it was like watching somebody going through all this process and I wasn't part of it. It was almost like I'd completely split so there was part of me voting and walking home, and there was the other part of me that wasn't there. But I could hear the doctor's words in my head, 'carcinoma'* [a type of cancer that starts in the skin or the lining of organs], *and that's all I heard. It went round in my head.*

Dee, breast cancer

First responses

Many people have a very clear memory of the moment they were given their diagnosis of cancer. For some, the diagnosis confirms what they have already been suspecting, while for others it comes like a bolt out of the blue. If you have been having symptoms investigated, cancer may have been on the list of possible causes. Screening programmes, such as those for breast and cervical screening, are designed specifically to detect abnormalities at an early stage – sometimes even before cancer actually develops. Being recalled after routine screening is bound to cause anxiety, even though identifying cancer at an early stage means treatment can be given when it is most likely to be curable. Occasionally cancer will be diagnosed as the result of investigations or treatment for a problem that seems completely unrelated.

No matter how prepared you may feel for a diagnosis of cancer, it will still come as a shock. Your reaction will be unique to you – people react in many different ways and there is no right or wrong way to respond. You may find yourself retreating into stunned silence, shock or disbelief. Or you may find yourself bursting into tears, feeling acutely distressed or blaming yourself. Anger is another common reaction. You will probably find that your responses change and you may experience all these reactions to some extent at one time or another. Again, it can be very helpful to understand there is no standard way to react. Once you have heard the word 'cancer' it can be difficult to take in anything else for some time.

Often it can be a relief knowing what is causing your symptoms, especially if they have been a problem for some time. Even so, this doesn't mean that you won't experience any of the reactions described above.

How the news is broken

The way in which people are told their diagnosis is just as important as the words used. Good communication is essential at this time, as it can set the tone of relationships between individuals and their health professionals for the future. Unfortunately, this is an area where some health professionals fall down. Many complaints made by patients and family members mention some sort of failure of communication. As one person points out:

> *There are huge differences in the experiences of patients being told bad news. Some doctors have made strenuous efforts to address this notoriously difficult area with further training. But others seem to think their practice is consummate when it is clear to the patient it is not. It is so obviously a training issue, but some at the top of their profession may see their training as complete. I wonder if the issue has become mingled for some with thoughts of omnipotence, especially since malignant tumours can be excised and lives can be saved.*
>
> **Mark, sarcoma**

Fortunately, there has now been widespread and official recognition that more training in communication skills is necessary for health professionals. Indeed, it is now recognised that the teaching of communication skills to student nurses and medical students should be given higher priority. The *NHS Cancer Plan* (see Chapter 2, pages 19–20) states that all cancer networks must draw up plans to provide training and support in communication skills for health professionals working in cancer units and centres. 'Bad news' can be any form of information that changes an individual's view of their future for the worse, and the professional's view of what this means may not always be the same as the patient's. Sensitivity and empathy are important. A situation where 'bad news' must be broken, can be made even more painful if handled insensitively. All cancer units and centres should have a policy for breaking bad news.

> *I found it shocking the way my consultant gave me my diagnosis and thought the way he told me did not allow me to ask any more about it. I had to accept the inevitable, instantly. I needed time to take it in, and he sat there staring at me. I managed to ask if my finger could be saved and he said it would flop around and get in the way. He offered no further explanation. I thought he wanted me to leave so he could deal with the other patients waiting outside. I wanted to know more, but he continued to stare at me, which I found very unnerving. I asked about a prosthesis for the metacarpal* [knuckle bone]. *He seemed a bit irritated at this and replied sharply, 'You're not listening to what I've said. You need to concentrate on the removal of the tumour in your hand.' I felt a strong reaction to this and*

blurted out, 'I am listening and it's my hand not yours.' He continued to stare at me.

Mark, sarcoma

Fortunately, not everyone has such a negative experience, as Dee found when she was diagnosed with breast cancer.

The breast care nurse was really good because she then went through the results in a language I could understand. She made it understandable, basically, she told me what the result was, what had happened and what was going to happen. It was distressing for me and she just said 'Let it out' and got lots of tissues and I just cried and cried.

Dee, breast cancer

Having someone with you

Ideally, you should be given the opportunity to have someone with you – a relative or friend – when you are given your diagnosis, and indeed for all health consultations. People are less likely to absorb and retain information when they are overwhelmed by life-changing news. This is one of the reasons why it can be helpful to have someone with you to act as a second pair of ears and eyes.

At the time of my diagnosis I was never asked if I wanted anyone with me. I was told late in the orthopaedic ward that the biopsy performed showed a malignant tumour. At the time, I had friends visiting and I was told to ask them to leave. I was not asked if I wanted to have anyone with me – a friend, a boyfriend or a partner or even my parents. I was given the news and then left alone. There are a lot of assumptions made by medical staff – it is important to state early on that if there is any unusual news you may or may not want someone with you.

Nina, sarcoma

Whether or not you have someone with you should be a matter of personal choice. Whereas some people find the presence of a trusted companion very helpful, others may have different preferences.

I know many people who would never attend a hospital appointment without being accompanied, but I prefer to go alone. It's bad enough for me to wait for ages, turning the pages of a book I'm not actually reading properly, but I don't want to have to cope with someone else's feelings. They have every right to be bored – I usually am, even though I'm so nervous – and I don't want to be responsible for that. After all, it's hardly the most appropriate venue for feeling that you have to keep people entertained!

Karen, breast cancer

Getting to grips with the language

If you have little experience of illness and hospitals, you will probably find some of the medical jargon difficult to understand at first. This can be very frustrating and may make you feel you have no control over the situation. But you will not be expected to have an immediate grasp of all the medical explanations and most people will not remember everything they are told. Doctors are trained as scientists and part of their training is to learn and understand technical terms. They don't always find it easy to explain medical information in terms that a non-medical person will understand. Your own background and experience will also affect how much technical information you want or are able to understand. Doctors (and other professionals) should try and pitch the information they are giving at a level that is right for you. But you may know better than they do what is appropriate, so be aware they may need your guidance about this. A good relationship with your doctor should make you feel sufficiently comfortable to say if you don't understand something. If you don't understand, perhaps you need to be given the information in a different way. Sometimes it can be easier to relate to other health professionals such as nurse specialists who may also be present when the diagnosis is given. Hearing the same information presented differently can often be easier to understand.

After tests had been done, my worst fear was realised. I was diagnosed with right breast carcinoma. I was told that the breast and all the axillary [underarm] nodes would have to be removed followed by chemotherapy, radiotherapy and then Tamoxifen for five years. Nothing really sunk in then. I did not know what these nodes were, what they did and what would be the result of their removal. I really didn't know what questions to ask. Realising now what these nodes do, I would have asked for some of them to remain if that were at all possible as I have now developed lymphoedema [swelling due to build up of lymphatic fluid in the tissues].

I was then seen by the Macmillan nurse. The last on the team but for me, she was the most important. I'm sure I would have fainted twice. Everything was gradually getting blacker and blacker and all I could hear was her voice talking to me softly, reassuring me and gradually bringing me back to the real world. Anytime I wanted to, she would speak to me on the phone or she would make an appointment for me to see her at the hospital. She really helped me to get through the initial stages of being told that I had breast cancer.

David, breast cancer

Communication problems can arise when information is presented in a form that is difficult to understand. Unfamiliar medical terms can be both difficult to understand and to remember. People are often reluctant to ask questions to clarify their understanding and doctors don't always check whether what they have said has been interpreted correctly and in context.

Writing in the *British Medical Journal* in 1995, a retired doctor provided the following illustration of how easy it can be to misinterpret language. During a recent hospital stay he found himself talking to a fellow patient who was clearly distressed. His wife had recently had a breast lump removed and the GP later called round to the house to give them the good news – that the lump was benign (non-cancerous). The GP then added 'So there's nothing more to be done about it – it's all finished' (meaning there was no further need for treatment as the problem had been dealt with). However, the couple had missed the satisfaction and relief shown by the doctor, hearing only the strange word 'benign' and that there was 'nothing more to be done'. This shows clearly that with information-giving, it is not just the words used but the meanings which the information-givers intend to convey and the inferences drawn by an individual that establishes their level of anxiety. People also interpret what they have been told within their own framework of ideas and theories of their illness.

Finding information

Even if initial test results indicate that you do have cancer, you may need further investigations before your doctor can discuss with you what sort of treatment you should have. This involves a period of uncertainty, which can give you a sense of being in limbo as you can't start planning your life to include treatment dates, for example. It does, however, give you the opportunity to think through some of the questions you might like to ask. One of the biggest problems here can be to know what questions you need to ask. Generally, we expect health professionals to provide the relevant information. But if information is not forthcoming, how can we know how much we don't yet know? (See pages 27–8 for some guidelines.)

How much do you want to know?

Think through how much you want to know about your illness. Do you want a lot of medical details now, or would it be easier just to have an overview for the time being? Knowing all the facts can help some people to feel more in control of what is happening to them. Others may find too much information unhelpful. Asking certain questions will not be at all straightforward, and it may help to spend a little time considering the impact of the various possible answers before you actually ask them.

Because most people find they have different information needs at different times, the questions they might benefit from most by asking around the time they first discover they have cancer are unlikely to be the same as the questions they will want or need the answers to at a later stage. A list of suggested additional questions that might be helpful for you to ask at the time you are diagnosed is given in Chapter 2, pages 27–8.

Initially, some people feel the question to which they most want an answer is, 'Am I going to die and, if so, when?' But this is a very difficult question to ask when you don't know if the answer will be something you can be happy about hearing. So, people ask less important questions instead, and find they can't listen to the answers. The time allowed for a consultation with the doctor or other health professionals is often too short, which can make people feel pressurised to try and achieve as much as possible in the time available. If you find yourself in this situation, you may well forget both what you are told, and what you wanted to ask. This is another reason for taking someone along with you.

I went in to hospital to have a cystoscopy [examination of the bladder] *and when I came out I was in complete agony. I couldn't walk, I couldn't move and I was really quite frightened so I rang up the hospital and they were clearly concerned. I said 'What's happening to me, can I come and see someone', thinking I needed some painkillers. So I went back to the hospital and in fact saw the surgeon. As I walked through the door he said to me 'Oh, it's cancer'. Not 'How are you, what's the problem' but 'It's cancer'. When I asked whether it was benign or malignant, the surgeon said 'It's malignant. We'll either take the lot out or you can have radiotherapy but we need to do some more tests'. I just looked at him and I said 'I can't take any more of this in.' The surgeon then said 'I'll make you another appointment for next week to come back and we'll talk some more and we'll organise all the tests'. I was just left in this complete vacuum. He just shunted me out of the consulting room and left. And that was probably one of the worst bits. I've said many times to other people about walking home in a bubble. I was in this complete bubble and I had to get home and I'd com-pletely forgotten to ask for any painkillers.*

Matthew, **bladder cancer**

A really empathetic health professional, on the other hand, can some-times anticipate exactly what a patient needs to know and when, as well as respond to questions. Sometimes, though, the doctor simply can't answer a patient's question. In such a case a doctor who is honest enough to admit this, rather than skating around the issue, is likely to gain much more trust and respect from the patient concerned.

The doctor was good. I could never understand what it was, these counts that people were looking for in my blood, and I could never really under-stand until this registrar explained it. What the markers [some cancers produce substances that can be monitored in the blood and these are known as tumour markers] *were and how they know if they're there. What I think you need to be clear about, and what doctors particularly don't tell you, is what they don't know. Actually, I've found that they've been quite good on the whole about telling me what they don't know. When you've really pushed them, they've said 'Well, we don't really know this'. That's why I can accept that.*

I need to know what the boundaries are. What I could know and what we can't know at the moment. Then I can stop worrying about it and I think I could deal much more effectively in every way – emotionally, physically with pain relief and everything – when I could understand the symptoms my body was giving out. Whether they're side effects of treatment, symp-toms actually of the cancer itself or post-operative things. Once I could understand what was causing those, I would know what to do about them.

Sadie, **colon cancer**

Reference

Symmers, W. StC. (1995) 'Explain in simple words – ensure the words are understood.' *British Medical Journal*, 310, page 1178.

Useful reading

C: Because Cowards Get Cancer Too (1999) John Diamond, Vermilion. ISBN: 0091816653

Cancer At Your Fingertips (2001) Val Speechley & Maxine Rosenfield, Class Publishing, London. ISBN: 1 85959 036 5

2
Finding your way around the cancer services

This chapter outlines what you can expect from the beginning of your 'cancer experience' and takes a look at current cancer services. It aims to give you a foundation from which you can build with blocks of information that will help you to understand and live with cancer.

Pre-diagnosis and diagnosis

The beginning of the 'cancer experience', for most people, is not the same as the moment they are given their diagnosis. Rather, this point may be confirmation of suspicions or symptoms that have been preoccupying them for some time. Indeed they may already have had an extremely unsettling period undergoing investigations for symptoms that may or may not turn out to be cancer.

How you are diagnosed will depend on where in the body the cancer starts. You may have had symptoms for a while, in which case the diagnosis may confirm what you have already suspected. Perhaps you attended a screening programme. A few people may learn they have cancer following investigations for other problems. Regardless of how your experience began, it is still going to come as a shock and you will be faced with an enormous learning curve. The whole consultation process itself can be overwhelming, particularly if your only experience of illness has been limited to the occasional visit to your GP.

So much has been said about cancer in the media, emphasizing prompt treatment, that people worry they won't be given enough time to think through the decisions they are being asked to make. On the other hand, time spent waiting for investigations and results can be equally stressful. Knowing what to expect at every stage, the timing of the investigations themselves and when you can expect to get the results will help you to cope during this period.

Pre-diagnosis is such a daunting part of the experience! All that unfamiliar equipment and strange procedures, and then there are the hospital staff to deal with. When they ask you to wait after the procedure and then pop their head round the door to say, 'That's absolutely fine, you can go now,' what are they telling you? We old hands know it only means that they've got what they need, which will be passed onto someone else for further investigation and an opinion. To patients with less experience it might signal 'All is well, you don't have cancer.' As a patient under investigation, you know full well that the technicians, who have looked at your scan to ensure that it's clear enough to help with a diagnosis, will have seen plenty of them before and have a good idea of what it shows. On one occasion I was stopped dead in my tracks when, as I was about to leave the department, the technician said, 'Good luck.' I interpreted it as meaning that she knew I'd need it! Somehow, the positive diagnosis a week later wasn't that much of a surprise.

Karen, breast cancer

The need for effective communication and good information can start way before the diagnosis is actually given. So how do you ensure, when you first notice that something isn't quite right, that you receive the appropriate investigations from the beginning?

An alien world

The medical world can seem a very alien place when you are suddenly thrown headlong into it. The unfamiliar language, strange environment and the different health professionals within the cancer team are all part of this new experience of living with cancer.

The term 'cancer' is itself one that carries many associations and misunderstandings. Often it is not until you experience cancer yourself (whether personally or through a family member or friend), that you realise what you do or don't know about the disease.

After I discovered a lump on my right breast in 1998, my GP told me that it was fat and would make an appointment at the hospital for it to be extracted. While waiting for this to be done, I picked up a Macmillan leaflet, which stated that 29,000 women and 206 men are diagnosed with breast cancer each year. It also gave the ten minimum standards of care for breast cancer. This was the first time I realised that men could have this

type of cancer and it sent a shiver through me. I wish I had known this before, as I would have been better prepared to receive the coming bad news.
David, breast cancer

There is so much to learn and understand about your illness, its treatment and how the health services work, that you may feel daunted by the whole process. This is where information can help you.

People have individual ways of coping with difficult news and it may take a while for the news to sink in. Some people find it is easier to imagine that what is happening to them is just a dream and that sooner or later they will wake up and life will be normal again. This reaction of disbelief has been likened to feeling that life is moving in slow motion. Others find that seeking out as much information as possible and talking to others in a similar situation is helpful to them. There is no right or wrong way to behave. What is too much information for one person may not be enough for another. You may experience a sense of panic that you need to have all the information straight away in order to feel in control of what's happening to you. It is unlikely that you will have to start making decisions immediately.

The role of your GP

Although one in three people in the UK will develop cancer at some stage in their lifetime, cancer forms a very small part of a GP's caseload. There are several reasons for this. Many other illnesses, for example, diabetes, heart disease, respiratory problems, are long term conditions and much of the treatment and care is managed by GPs in between hospital visits. With cancer, however, treatment is normally given in hospital and it is the hospital health professionals who provide most of the care during a course of treatment. Many people, once their treatment has finished are able to resume their regular lives, only going back to the hospital for regular check-ups. GPs will see on average, about eight new diagnoses of cancer a year. Even the more common cancers are regarded as rare. The geographical area of a GP practice is another factor influencing how many people with cancer will be seen by the doctor. Cancer is a disease that affects mainly older people. Practices with a higher percentage of older people will see more people with cancer than practices with a younger population.

GPs clearly have an important role in identifying symptoms of suspected cancers and knowing when to refer on to diagnostic and specialist services. To help GPs, there are national guidelines for the urgent referral of patients with suspected cancer. The *Referral Guidelines for Suspected*

Cancer (DoH, 2000) help GPs identify those people who are most likely to have cancer and who should be referred on to a specialist. They can also help identify people who are unlikely to have cancer and require non-urgent referral to hospital. A specialist should see anyone with symptoms that may suggest cancer, within two weeks of their GP making a referral. There are no common symptoms of cancer. It is the combination of symptoms along with factors such as age and gender, as well as risk factors for the relevant cancer such as smoking and family history, that alert doctors to the possibility of cancer.

I knew I was ill a long time before I did anything about it. I always thought I was the sort who would immediately go straight to my doctor. I'd never been able to really understand people who said they were ill and put off going to the doctor and I never would have thought I'd be that sort of person. Having a major illness was just not on my agenda. I just didn't have time to fit in something like cancer. I think subconsciously that's what was going on. Every time I went to the loo for about seven months, I said I must go to the doctor and every time I said I'll do it next week, it's probably only a polyp. I went to see my GP, who was appalled because things were getting quite pressing by that time and I was getting quite a lot of symptoms. Not enough to interfere with my life but enough to make things a bit uncomfortable. She behaved as though it was a very urgent problem and I would be seen immediately. She didn't commit herself and said it could be anything. Yes, it could be cancer, it could be diverticulitis – I didn't know what that was – it could be irritable bowel, it could be anything. In the event I waited ten weeks for an appointment at the hospital, by which time I was getting very uncomfortable indeed and quite frightened because things over that last two months really got a lot worse.

Sadie, colon cancer

Different ways of managing cancer

The diagnosis and treatment of cancer depends on the type of cancer and where it started in the body. Different cancers behave in different ways and therefore, they may be managed in a number of ways. This process is often described as a cancer pathway. You may find that you have tests and follow-up appointments in your local hospital but then have to travel to a different hospital for treatment.

As cancer can occur anywhere in the body, it is easier to think in terms of groups of cancers, relating to the different areas of the body. They are:

- Lung cancer

- Upper gastrointestinal cancers (oesophagus, stomach, pancreas)

- Lower gastrointestinal cancers (colon or bowel, rectum)

- Breast cancer

- Gynaecological cancers (ovary, uterus, cervix)

- Urological cancers (bladder, kidney, prostate, testis – the last two are sometimes grouped together as 'men's cancers')

- Haematological malignancies (leukaemia, non-Hodgkin's lymphoma, Hodgkin's disease, myeloma)

- Skin cancers (melanoma)

- Head and neck cancers (mouth, lip, pharynx, larynx, thyroid)

- Brain/central nervous system tumours

- Sarcomas (soft tissue, bone)

- Children's tumours

It will depend on the type of cancer your GP thinks you may have as to which hospital specialist you will be referred to. If, for instance, you had problems with swallowing, you might be referred to a gastroenterologist or if you had problems with your breathing, to a chest physician. Not all symptoms are easy to diagnose. Some people go to their GP with non-specific symptoms such as tiredness resulting from anaemia and may well be referred to a general physician for an initial assessment. Once the cause of the anaemia is found, then a referral should be made to the appropriate specialist.

Not every patient will be referred in this way. Sometimes cancers are discovered at an early stage when a person is having treatment for a problem which may be unrelated. Some people learn they have cancer following an emergency admission to hospital, providing no time for any preparation for the diagnosis to come.

The symptoms I had, which I now know but I didn't realise at the time, were because it was bladder cancer. I was passing a lot of urine and blood so I didn't go my GP. I went to the urinary clinic at the hospital because it was the waterworks department. I thought they'd probably know more than going to the GP. The doctor said 'Well I don't know what it is, we'll give you these pills, some antibiotics and come back in two weeks'. So the following week I began passing blood clots and I thought this is not on so I went back. About two days later, I went to the A & E and I sat on a trolley for three hours and I explained I'd got an appointment with the urologist but it wasn't for two or three weeks. They said we can't get you in any earlier but what we can do is do some of the tests before you go. That was quite positive but it was very strange because I suddenly had to take charge of part of my life that I hadn't done before. I was battling against the establishment as it were. I'd been pushed onto this very slow conveyor belt.

Matthew, bladder cancer

Overwhelming though it might seem in itself, the diagnosis of cancer is often part of a rather less dramatic process. Indeed, many people are diagnosed as a result of having attended a screening programme. Currently breast screening (mammogram) is available three-yearly to all women between the ages of 50 and 64. This programme will be extended to all women aged 65–70 by 2004 and screening will be available on request to women over 70. The cervical screening programme offers a smear test to all women aged 20 to 64 at least once every five years. Other programmes that may be introduced in the future if pilot studies prove successful include screening all people aged 50–69 for colorectal (bowel) cancers, ovarian cancer screening for women and the PSA test to detect prostate cancer in men. PSA – short for prostate specific antigen – is a chemical produced by the prostate gland and released into the bloodstream. The PSA test measures the levels of this chemical in the blood. Although it may be raised if there is benign (non-cancerous) enlargement of the prostate gland, it is usually higher if cancer is present.

Many people will find that their cancer care is shared between more than one hospital. While it is often more convenient to receive treatment in a local hospital, you may find that you have to travel to another hospital for specialist tests or treatment.

The *NHS Cancer Plan*

One of the first questions many people ask is, 'Am I being treated in the right place by the right people?' Cancer care and treatment has been likened to a postcode lottery. So much has depended on where an individual lives and the local services available to them. To ensure that everyone has access to good cancer services, the Department of Health (DoH) published the *NHS Cancer Plan* in 2000. It sets out, for the first time, a

programme of how cancer services should be managed in England, bringing together prevention, diagnosis, treatment, care and research.

The *NHS Cancer Plan* is being put into action through 34 cancer networks in England. Each cancer network brings together all the organisations that have an interest in cancer. These include strategic health
authorities, hospitals, community health services, the voluntary organisations and local authorities. The number of hospital trusts varies
between each network, depending on the geographical area. The networks provide three levels of care. *Primary care* refers to medical care provided in the community. This is delivered by Primary Care Trusts (PCTs),
which consist of GP (family doctor) practices and community health services. PCTs are responsible for the planning and obtaining of health services and improving the health of the local population.

Cancer Units, which are found in most hospitals, have the expertise and
facilities to treat the more common cancers. *Cancer Centres* provide expertise in the management of all cancers, both common and rare. These are

Cancer Network

Cancer Centre
Usually a teaching hospital (there are some joint cancer centres
with 2 or 3 hospitals) providing expertise in the management of
all cancers which provide specialist services such as radiotherapy

Cancer Support Centres
These are usually community-
based, voluntary organisations

Primary Care Trusts
GP (family doctor) practices and
community health services

Cancer Units
Local hospitals (there may be
any number between 2–15),
which have the expertise and
facilities to treat the more
common cancers

usually based in teaching hospitals and provide specialist services such as radiotherapy. They are also likely to carry out research and education. In some cancer networks, there may be two hospitals coming together to form a joint Cancer Centre. For every Cancer Centre, there will be several Cancer Units.

It is through cancer networks that all aspects of cancer services can be planned across the care pathway – prevention, screening, diagnosis, treatment, supportive care and specialist palliative care. Cancer services are being redesigned so that everyone has the opportunity to receive a consistent quality of treatment and care.

The Department of Health (DoH) has published several documents to help put the Cancer Plan into practice. One of the best ways of finding out about them is through the DoH website (see page 151). You can also obtain copies through the post by writing to them.

It has been clearly shown that a co-ordinated team of health professionals who have interest and expertise in a particular cancer should be providing treatment and care. Health professionals are only going to gain experience when they see sufficient numbers of people with the same type of cancer. Most hospitals see enough people with the more common cancers such as breast, lung and bowel cancers, to have Cancer Units with the staff and facilities to ensure high quality diagnosis, treatment and care. The smaller number of people with rarer cancers, sarcomas for example, means they are likely to get better care by going to a hospital that sees larger numbers, usually a Cancer Centre.

It is important to find out if there are any centres that specialise in your form of cancer. For example with a rare cancer like a sarcoma I later discovered the Middlesex specialised in this form. It would've helped me feel less isolated during and after my treatment if I had been in touch with other similar cases.

Nina, sarcoma

While you may be diagnosed and receive treatment at your local hospital, for more specialised cancer treatments such as radiotherapy and bone marrow transplantation, you will need to go to a Cancer Centre. As many cancer specialists from the Cancer Centres run outpatient clinics in the Cancer Units, you will often be able to have follow-up appointments locally. One of the most important functions of the cancer networks is to bring together all these different services so that the care you receive is co-ordinated.

Cancer Services Collaborative

The Cancer Services Collaborative is a national programme working with cancer networks across the country to make the way cancer care is managed more efficient. They are looking at ways to improve local services from the moment an individual is referred for diagnosis onwards. Through the cancer networks, services can be planned in the most effective way to meet the needs of people in any given area. In the third phase of the Cancer Services Collaborative (starting in 2003) Service Improvement Facilitators will work with the local cancer health professionals to help them to review and improve the current patient experience.

Part of the work carried out by the Cancer Services Collaborative is to look at patients' experience and highlight where improvements can be made. Already it is quite clear that the organisation of investigations could be streamlined to avoid individuals having to attend a hospital on several different occasions. While this can be very trying, it doesn't help when people forget to cancel an appointment they can't make. Let the hospital know if you can't keep an appointment and remember to let them know if you change your name, address, telephone number or GP.

Timekeeping

The experience of having to wait for out-patient appointments, investigations or treatment can be very frustrating. Hospitals are trying various ways to deal with this. Some clinics and departments have introduced ticket systems, similar to those in supermarkets, and this can give you a better idea of how long you may have to wait. A common worry when waiting is often 'Have I got time to buy a drink or go to the loo?' It is always worth asking the reception staff, as they should have a good idea of what the waiting times are likely to be. You can help yourself, as well, by bringing a book to read or something to occupy you. You may want to mention how long you have had to wait, and find out what can be done to improve things (see Chapter 9).

The cancer team

If you have had very little experience of hospitals you may find meeting different health professionals for the first time rather daunting. If you don't know what their role is, it is very difficult to recognise how they can help you with specific questions or practical problems.

The rest of this chapter is designed to give you an idea of who the different people you may come across within the cancer team may be and what their roles are.

Medical specialists

As mentioned earlier in this chapter, it will depend on the type of cancer your GP thinks you may have as to which hospital specialist you will be referred to. Once your cancer has been diagnosed, you may then be referred on to a cancer specialist. As more than one type of treatment is often used, you may find that several specialist doctors are involved in your care. These are the specialists you may meet:

- Cancer surgeons

- Clinical oncologists

- Haematologists

- Medical oncologists

- Palliative medicine consultants

Consultants are hospital specialists. They have completed specialist training and are in overall charge and supervise the work of a team of doctors including specialist registrars, senior house officers and house officers.

Cancer surgeons

Cancer surgeons carry out operations to remove tumours (cancer growths). A cancer surgeon specialises in a particular part of the body, such as the bowel or the lungs. As well as having an interest and experience in cancer surgery, they may also carry out non-cancer surgery.

Clinical oncologists

Clinical oncologists treat cancer with radiotherapy treatments (high energy x-rays). Most clinical oncologists will also prescribe chemotherapy (anti-cancer drugs) and hormone therapies. They usually specialise in treating particular types of cancer.

Haematologists

Haematologists are specialists in diagnosing and treating blood disorders. These include cancers such as leukaemias (affecting the bone marrow), lymphomas (affecting lymphatic tissue) and myelomas (affecting the plasma cells in the bone marrow).

Medical oncologists

Medical oncologists treat cancer with drugs. These include chemotherapy, biological therapies and hormone therapies. Like clinical oncologists, they usually specialise in treating particular types of cancer.

Palliative medicine consultants

Palliative medicine consultants are specialists in the management of pain and other physical symptoms caused by the cancer or side effects of the treatment. They also care for the emotional, social and spiritual needs of individuals and their families.

Other health professionals

You are likely to come into contact with a number of other health-related professionals who make up the cancer team. Although you are most likely to meet them in hospital, you may meet some of these professionals in other settings such as the community or in local hospices.

These are the professionals you may meet:

- Appliance officer
- Chaplain
- Counsellor
- Dietitian
- Occupational therapist
- Physiotherapist
- Radiographer
- Social work team
- Specialist cancer nurse
- Speech and language therapist

Appliance officer

The appliance officer can provide a variety of services. In some hospitals it is the appliance officer who will fit breast prostheses following surgery (rather than a breast care nurse) and advise on swimwear, sundresses and nightwear. If your treatment is likely to cause hair loss, they can supply wigs. The appliance officer may fit compression stockings or tights, for individuals with swollen limbs.

Chaplain

We all have a spiritual dimension and while for some people religion or other faith is an important part of spiritual care, for others it is not. While most hospitals provide a chaplain from the Christian church, more hospitals and hospices are providing chaplains from other faiths and will be happy to send for a representative of any religion or faith. However, you don't have to have any particular faith or beliefs to talk to a member of the chaplaincy team. They are also there to help you talk through questions like 'Why me?'

Counsellor

Many people say that they experienced a whole range of different emotions when they were given their cancer diagnosis. While you may feel you can talk to your family and or friends, some people find it helpful to talk to someone who is specially trained. Some cancer departments have trained counsellors or psychotherapists with whom you can discuss things.

Dietitian

Difficulties with eating due to problems such as loss of appetite, a sore mouth or taste changes can be a result of both the cancer and its treatment. As good nutrition will help you to recover more quickly, you may find it helpful to talk to a dietitian who can offer advice on how to overcome these problems, including nutritional supplements if they are appropriate. They can also advise on how to eat healthily following treatment and answer questions about whether to take vitamin and mineral supplements and other nutritional approaches to cancer. There are also community-based dietitians, working outside hospitals.

Occupational therapist

If you find it difficult to manage at home because of practical difficulties, occupational therapists (OTs) can assess your needs to help you become as independent as possible. They can assess how you manage in your home and advise if any equipment or adaptations could help you. They can also help with teaching you other ways of managing activities such as washing, dressing and cooking. Occupational therapists also work outside hospitals and clinics, coming to your home.

Physiotherapist

There are a number of ways in which physiotherapy can help to maintain or improve your physical fitness. Physiotherapists can help prevent and treat breathing difficulties after surgery and advise on exercises after treatment. They can also assess your mobility and physical needs, and provide equipment such as sticks, crutches and frames to help with walking. Community-based physiotherapists will visit you at home.

Radiographer

Radiographers are trained to work with x-rays and radioactive substances. There are two different types of radiographer: diagnostic radiographers and therapeutic radiographers.

You will meet diagnostic radiographers if you have any investigations such as x-rays, CT scans or ultrasound scans.

Therapeutic radiographers work in radiotherapy departments and are the main people you will come into contact with when you have radiotherapy treatment. They help plan and give your treatment and will be able to answer many of your questions. They are also able to advise on possible side effects and what you can or can't do during treatment.

Social work team

Social workers are experienced in working with people who have to adjust to change or crisis in their lives. They can provide information and advise on community services to support you when you go home. They work closely with the social service teams in the community who will be able to arrange for any help you may need at home. Some hospitals have a Welfare Rights Adviser who can give you information and advice on housing, employment and immigration issues, welfare benefits and financial difficulties.

Specialist cancer nurse

Like doctors, many nurses specialise in different areas of cancer care. This may be in a particular type or group of cancers such as the specialist nurse in urology who works with people with bladder, kidney and prostate cancers. Other specialist nurses may work in a particular area of care such as chemotherapy, symptom control or palliative care, lymphoedema (see page 10) and emotional support. In some hospitals, especially the Cancer Centres, you may come into contact with research nurses. You will meet them if you are invited to take part in a clinical trial and they will discuss the details of the trial with you and support you throughout if you decide to go ahead.

Specialist cancer nurses may also be known as clinical nurse specialists and Macmillan Nurses. You will meet specialist cancer nurses in hospitals, hospices and the community.

Speech and language therapist

Speech therapists provide practical help for people who have developed difficulties with communication and/or swallowing as a result of their cancer or its treatment. There are also community-based speech therapists.

How do I get in contact with these people?

It depends on the type of cancer and treatment you have as to which of these health professionals you will come into contact with. Some you will meet before your treatment and some you may meet afterwards. It can be very helpful to have a specialist nurse with you when you are first told you have cancer, especially if you want to ring up later on to ask any questions that may occur to you after getting home. It is also helpful to know what arrangements have been made for holiday/sickness cover and who you can contact in the absence of the person you would normally see. Ask your hospital doctor or specialist nurse to make arrangements if you wish to see any member of the cancer team.

'Getting the best from your cancer services: questions for patients to ask'

The Commission for Health Improvement (CHI) and the Audit Commission undertook a large study of cancer services *NHS Cancer Care in England and Wales*, published in December 2001. They have produced a leaflet from the report called 'Getting the best from your cancer services: Questions for Patients to Ask' (also referred to in Chapter 5, pages 58–9). The questions have been divided into three sections – diagnosis, treatment and care and palliative care. After each question they've described the features of a good service to help you understand what should happen at each stage. See *Resources* at the end of this chapter for details of how to order a copy.

The questions listed overleaf are ones you may wish to ask when you are being diagnosed.

Questions to ask your GP

- What are you referring me to a consultant for?

- How quickly will I be seen? Are you referring me as 'urgent' or 'non urgent'?

- How long will it be before I have all the tests? Where will they be carried out? Will I need to visit several departments?

- What are the tests for? How many will I need? Who will give me the results and when?

- Will the person doing the test look after me while it is being done? Will they tell me what to expect?

- What times are available for me to have my tests, for instance, could they be done in the evening?

- Is the doctor I will be seeing a recognised cancer specialist?

- Will the doctor have all my test results? Will the meeting be for diagnosis or treatment?

- Can I bring someone with me to discuss my diagnosis and treatment?

- Will the consultant understand my concerns and give me time to ask questions? Will a specialist nurse be there to help me?

Questions to ask at the hospital

- Who can I telephone when I think of questions later? Can I make another appointment to see someone in person? Can I seek a second opinion?

- Will someone have passed on the diagnosis and information about the treatments planned to my GP? How quickly will this happen?

Resources

Cancer Research UK
PO Box 123, Lincoln's Inn Fields, London WC2A 3PX
Tel: 0800 226 237 *or* 020 7061 8355
www.cancerhelp.org.uk

Government documents about cancer services can be found on the Department of Health website at: www.doh.gov.uk/cancer

General information on specific cancers and on issues surrounding cancer can be found on: www.royalmarsden.org and www.cancerbacup.org.uk

The CancerBACUP Helpline number is 0808 800 1234

The leaflet 'Getting the best from your cancer services: Questions for Patients to Ask' can be downloaded free from: www.chi.nhs.uk or from www.audit-commission.gov.uk or ordered from The Stationery Office on 0870 600 5522.

More advice on how to gain information can be found in Chapter 10

3
Communicating with the health professionals

Good communication with your doctor and other health professionals is terribly important. We all communicate in different ways and will relate to some people better than others. Not trusting or liking the person you're dealing with can be a barrier to good communication. You may prefer your doctor to treat you as an equal partner when making decisions about your future. Or you may prefer to see your doctor as the 'medical expert' who will make decisions for you. Most people value those doctors who listen to them, and who place equal importance on emotional needs as well as medical needs.

There is much that you can do to get the best out of your relationship with your health professionals. While many doctors are good communicators, communication is a two-way process and you also have a responsibility to keep them informed. Doctors and other health professionals need you to tell them how you are feeling and what difficulties you may be experiencing. They are not mind readers. There are many reasons why you may feel reluctant to talk about your feelings, anxieties or problems. When clinics or GP surgeries are busy, you may feel there isn't enough time at your appointment to go through everything that's on your mind.

It is very important that your doctor knows what your symptoms are, and you have a part to play in ensuring that the information you give is as full and accurate as possible. You may find it helpful (indeed, so may your doctor) to prepare a written list of symptoms and a note of the times they appear and any other significant circumstances. Keeping a 'symptom diary' is one way of producing an accurate account, for example.

Embarrassment can sometimes make it difficult to 'open up'. Often people assume that doctors and other health professionals working in this field will know how they must be feeling. There may be an expectation that the doctor will ask the appropriate questions to find out how you are feeling or if you have any problems. Perhaps you think your problem is too trivial or it's a reflection on your ability to cope. Coming to terms with a life threatening disease is not something most people have had to adjust to before. Therefore the normal coping mechanisms that usually work well in other situations may not work so well here. It may not be easy talking about feelings if you don't generally share your feelings with other people. It can be uncomfortable voicing thoughts that you would prefer to keep at the back of your mind.

> *The first operation was a lumpectomy, they just took the lump out and then they did a biopsy. You have the week of not knowing the result. There was this part of me that was just thinking everything's going to be all right, because everybody kept saying everything will be all right, and I really believed everything was fine. I had to go back as an outpatient for the results. They said that there were lots of cancer cells in the breast still, they'd removed all the lymph nodes and there was one that was affected. He (the surgeon) kept saying that this is good and that I must hold onto that. I still kept thinking 'I'm going to die' and I remember him saying it costs a lot of money to treat someone with cancer with operations and chemo and if the prognosis wasn't good we wouldn't go through all this trouble basically. He didn't put it like that, but that's what he meant.*
>
> **Dee, breast cancer**

Another reason for not telling your doctor about something that's bothering you is the fear of what it could mean. Often you will find that you have been worrying unnecessarily. However, if it turns out that your fears are real, then the earlier your doctor knows about the problem, the earlier the opportunity to do something about it. Talking to a member of your health care team about how you are feeling may lead to the reassurance that your difficulties are a common experience and to finding out that there are ways of helping you through them.

Your relationship with your doctor

Perhaps it is difficult to like someone who is giving you news that turns your world upside down. On the other hand, the doctor might be seen as a saviour, the hope for a future. We choose our friends from the many people we meet throughout our life. Not everyone we meet will become a friend. Just because we wouldn't want to socialise with some individuals doesn't mean we don't have respect for them. In the same way, you may not instantly feel a rapport with your doctor. Communication is a two way process and misunderstandings happen because one or both participants fail to be clear in the messages they give. If you are not naturally assertive, you may perhaps be afraid of seeming to be too demanding, or of seeming foolish because you don't understand what you're being told. Shock at what you're being told can often lead to all the questions you want to ask flying out of the window. When you are given unwelcome information, it can be helpful when doctors allow you to express your feelings. It can take time to work through your feelings and you may find it helpful to talk to someone else at this stage, perhaps a counsellor or someone who has been through a similar experience (see Chapter 7).

Or you may not yet feel ready to take in all the information you are being given – so you may become distressed by it or simply not hear it. Sometimes you will need to come back and seek out information you have already been given, but not absorbed, at a later stage.

Find a way of communicating with your doctor that feels right for you. Communication can be face to face, by letter or fax, or take the form of a telephone conversation. Modern technology has opened up new channels of communication such as e-mail, although this won't suit everyone – either individuals or doctors!

> *I still had lots of questions after I had seen the first surgeon. After agonising about what to do (surgery was just two weeks away), I decided to write to him with my e-mail address and fax details on the top of the letter. He replied by fax and said that we could correspond by e-mail. We then had several exchanges in the next few days, which were just what I needed to sort out all my questions before the surgery. I was blessed that he was very experienced with e-mail. The surgeon from whom I had sought a second opinion gave me a card with his e-mail address on it, but never replied to my subsequent e-mail to him.*
>
> **Ellen, breast cancer**

For the relationship to work, it must be a two-way exchange of information. Remember that doctors aren't mind readers so you will have to tell them how you feel. Make a note (for example in a notebook kept expressly for this purpose, or a 'symptom diary') of any symptoms you have to tell the doctor on your next visit. Don't assume that they are unimportant and not worth mentioning. Any physical changes are bound to cause anxiety and if it turns out that they are not significant, your mind can be put at rest. Being honest about lifestyle habits such as smoking may not be easy, but all information helps the doctor to develop a clearer picture about you. This will ensure that you receive the right treatment and care.

I was referred to a general physician, a consultant physician, and if I had known that I was going to see anybody as marvellous as she was, and as nice and as sort of gentle and understanding, I would have gone months before.

Sadie, colon cancer

It can also be helpful to talk to your doctor about the impact of cancer on your lifestyle. Think about what is most important to you, and ask your specialist how these aspects are likely to be affected by the disease and its treatment. For example, do you work or are you self-employed? Perhaps you have young children, or care for an older relative or friend, or you live alone. Not everyone lives near the hospital where they will receive treatment and travelling may cause additional anxiety. Telling your doctor how you feel can open the door to other sources of help during this difficult time.

Two days after [being given my diagnosis – see page 8], *I contacted my local cancer resource centre. I discovered they offered counselling and I made a booking. Within a week I was sitting with a counsellor addressing my anger and frustration as well as describing the healing conversations I'd had at home. My GP was prepared to discuss my experience with me too. I was able to come to terms with the diagnosis and how it had been delivered in a short time, thanks to a positive approach within my family and professionals I sought out for myself. I am not lucky; I should not have been faced with crass insensitivity and ignorance of the patient's needs in the first place.*

Mark, sarcoma

Barriers to communication

The time around diagnosis can highlight potential barriers to good communication. While they are not exclusive to diagnosis and can be a concern at any stage of the illness, it may be helpful to outline the major barriers here:

- Fear of the unknown;

- Uncertainty about how much information you can cope with;

- Remembering what you have been told;

- Knowing what questions you want to ask;

- Understanding what you have been told;

- Feeling under pressure to make immediate decisions.

Overcoming barriers to communication

There are ways of overcoming these barriers. These are some of the things that people have found useful:

- Talking through your questions with a friend so that you are clearer about what you need to know and what information will be most useful to you;

- Writing down the questions you want to ask, so that you will not forget them when you are actually with the doctor;

- Taking someone with you when you are seeing the doctor or any health professional;

- Deciding on one or two important questions and leaving others until later;

- Being aware that the doctor may also find it hard;

- Thinking about how you would deal with different answers to a question before you ask it;

- Repeating back what you think you've heard, to check you've got it right;

- Remembering that you are the 'service user' and the job of the health professional is to provide you with the information you need.

Some people have said that they were not given the opportunity to ask questions or that health professionals seemed reluctant to share their information. They may have felt '*fobbed off*' by health professionals when given a very medical response. Sometimes doctors think they have covered everything and assume you will ask questions if need be. It is easy to forget that what is so familiar to health professionals because they are working in the field is perhaps new to the person sitting in front of them.

The following strategies are ones you may find helpful when you visit your doctor.

Before your appointment

Length of time of a consultation

The average time allowed for an appointment is often only 5 to 10 minutes. In order to make the best possible use of the time allocated to you, you could start by asking the receptionist how long your next appointment is expected to last. Then you can prepare beforehand so that you are better able to achieve what you want to achieve in that time. Feeling rushed during a consultation can be just as frustrating for health professionals as it is for you. Remember that communication is a two-way process and think about what information your doctor may need from you. You can make better use of the time if you have already made notes about, for example, symptoms you have been experiencing. You may find it helpful to write down a list of symptoms and the dates when you first noticed them (keeping a 'symptom diary' – see page 32).

> *It is an excellent idea to make a list in advance of the things you want to discuss in the consultation – it's a well known fact that most of us seem to abandon our brains at the hospital entrance! It's no good thinking that, if it's important enough, you'll remember to ask, because you probably won't. I've never encountered a doctor who had a problem with lists. On the contrary, I get the impression that they appreciate patients who try to be organised and make the most of their consultation time.*
>
> **Karen, breast cancer**

The length of time allowed will also depend on the reason for the consultation. When the purpose of the consultation is to give you your diagnosis, generally doctors try to ensure that they allow sufficient uninterrupted time.

People are often reluctant to ask questions for fear of taking up the doctor's valuable time, especially when they know the clinic is busy. Or they may fear that the question they want to ask will appear stupid. No question is stupid or not worth asking. Health professionals will not think any the less of you for your questions, and the chances are that asking them will save you unnecessary worry. As your time with the doctor will be limited, it may be helpful to ask the questions that are most important to you before you leave. If you still have any unanswered questions, either request another appointment or find out whether anyone else can answer them.

How much information do you want?

Without necessarily knowing what your doctor is going to tell you, it can be helpful to think about how much information you feel you can cope with at any one time. Tell your doctor what kind of information you want and in how much detail. This way, you will feel you have some control during the consultation.

I went to the hospital with a friend, expecting the doctor to tell me that I had cancer. I'd already got a list of questions I was going to ask, almost on the assumption I was going to be told that I had cancer or certainly knowing that I was going to have an operation. At that stage, I knew that I would need information, practical things like would I be able to go on the holiday I'd booked and how much time would I need off work. The first thing I wanted to know really about cancer, was 'What's the prognosis, am I going to die?' The consultant said to me 'You've got cancer'. And that was what I'd expected to hear but she was very, very good and she gave me a lot of time. She said 'I know that when you go to see the surgeon tomorrow, he won't be able to give you this amount of time because I've fitted you into his clinic so I'll answer any questions I can'. And she was very clear in so far as she could be about the information and she said that 95% of people who get through five years have no further problem. She said 'You've got a lot to be positive about'. And that was very important, something I hung on to.

Sadie, colon cancer

Talking through your questions

It may be useful to map out, by talking to a family member or friend or using pencil and paper, the areas that you are unclear about. Maybe they can ask you questions about things that they don't understand: this may prompt you to realise that it is also a question for you. Don't feel you have to think of all the possible questions at this stage. There will be plenty of other times when you will be able to ask questions.

The first time I was diagnosed with cancer, a good friend opened a decent bottle of wine, handed me a notepad and pen and said, 'Right, have a drink and make a list.' You have no idea how much that helped. In a frantic brain-storming session I wrote down everything I wanted to attend to before going into hospital for surgery. By the time the bottle was empty I'd got a prioritised list, which proved invaluable over the next few days. Apart from the friend who helped me to get focused, nobody knew what to make of my initial reactions. I rushed off to make a new will, got all my paperwork in order and tidied all the drawers and cupboards. Organisation was my watchword! I've been diagnosed with cancer twice more since then and, on each occasion, have instinctively repeated this pattern of behaviour. I know now that I felt as though my life was running out of control, so I tried to get that control back in any areas I could.

Karen, breast cancer

Writing questions down
Writing a question down can help to make it clearer to you what it is you really want to know. You can look at what you have written the next day to see if it is still the question you want to ask.

Deciding on one or two important questions
It isn't easy to take in a lot of new information at one time, so it may be useful to think of the most important questions and to ask these first. In this way, you have a better chance of remembering what you have been told. The answers to these questions may then prompt you to think of more questions.

Taking someone with you
Just as some people would welcome more information at the beginning, equally there are others who feel that they have been given too much information. One solution adopted by many people is to take a family member or friend to consultations when they knew they are likely to be *'overwhelmed'* or *'bombarded'* with information. They can offer you moral support, remind you of questions you wanted to ask and listen to what you are being told so that you get another view of what was said.

Thinking about how you would deal with different answers to a question before you ask it
There are some questions (for example, 'Should I give up smoking?') that you probably know the answer to already. Ask yourself what your response would be to the answer 'Yes' or the answer 'No'.

There is other, more complex, information that you don't have, but could still begin to map out some response to, such as 'When will I get back to work?' The doctor may say, for example, 'We don't know yet until we see how you respond to the treatment' or alternatively 'In six (or nine) months time'. Imagine how you might deal with the different possible information you may get. This can make it easier to understand what is being said to you and to think of further information that you may need. Often people find that, with time, they become more confident in asking questions and knowing what information could be helpful.

Questions about prognosis can be difficult to ask when the answers could be difficult to hear. You may feel you can only ask them once you are ready to deal with possible answers.

Remembering that you are the 'service user' and the job of the health professional is to provide you with the information you need

It is often easy to feel intimidated or worried about seeming awkward. It can be useful to remember that health professionals are increasingly aware of people's need for clear, accurate, timely and relevant information. More to the point, it is now a part of their job to provide this. If you see yourself as a service user rather than as a patient, it may be easier to feel entitled to good information.

So I went home and thought about it, and phoned an old friend I hadn't seen for years, and she made an appointment for me to go and see a radiotherapist she worked with. He was quite, quite different and he treated me quite differently from the surgeon, like a proper person with a mind.

Anne, breast cancer

Ask what happens next

Before you leave the building, make sure you know what the next step will be – another appointment, a course of treatment or whatever. Make sure you are not left in the air.

During your appointment

The presence of other people

Ideally, when you are given your diagnosis or any unwelcome news, an appropriate specialist nurse should be present with the doctor. This can be helpful if you then see the nurse at a later time, as they will know exactly what information you were given during the consultation. While you may have chosen to take a family member or friend with you to your appointment, you may find that the presence of other health professionals makes you feel uncomfortable. Your doctor should always introduce other health professionals who are in the room and, if medical students are present, ask if you mind them being there. Don't feel you that you have to agree if you would prefer to see the doctor on your own. There may also be times when you want an opportunity to talk to the doctor without the person who is accompanying you being present.

Writing down information

Just as it can be helpful to write down questions before your appointment, it can be helpful to write down some of the information that is given to you during it. People often find that once they get back home, they can't remember everything (or even anything) that was said. Writing down information such as what investigations you will need and the dates and times, if known, will help back up your memory. You may also find it helpful to make a note of the treatment proposed for you, such as the names of any drugs, and the names of the key health professionals you will come into contact with. It can also be useful to note down how to contact them.

> *I used to write and I kept a notebook from day one. Every time I went to see someone about a test or a result or something, this notebook came along and anything was written down. So I was able to write down things before I went to see them, questions that I had because I knew, like most people, that once you get in there, your mind just goes a complete blank. Also, at the very beginning it was quite stressful and usually one of my friends came with me. I found that very helpful because although I had questions to ask, they sometimes had questions that I hadn't thought about.*
>
> **Matthew, bladder cancer**

Tape-recording the consultation

You might want to consider taking along a tape recorder to the consultation as this is another way of recalling the discussion between you and your doctor. It can help to refresh your memory and you may hear new information that you don't remember hearing the first time round. Some people say that they find it useful to listen to audiotapes of consultations with other family members who were unable to be with them at the consultation.

However, you may find that your doctor is reluctant to allow you to tape the interview. Even if it is agreed that the interview be taped, you may find your doctor becomes more cautious about giving certain information while the machine is turned on.

Distressing information

Many people say that it's hard to retain unwelcome or upsetting information and that they will forget some of it as a way of protecting themselves.

It can be helpful asking for the same information more than once, as each time you receive it you are likely to understand and remember a little bit more.

Finding out who can provide further information between appointments
There is a huge amount of information to absorb, particularly when you are first given your diagnosis. This is likely to mean that you won't be able to think of all the questions at the one time. It is important to find out who you can talk to in between appointments if you do have further questions, and how you can contact them.

> *Nothing had prepared me for the overwhelming power of fear and uncertainty that the news of having secondary cancer brought. I felt as though I was being crushed between two uncontrollable forces. Firstly the cancer inside me that seemed to be growing rapidly and secondly the onslaught of well meaning but confusing medical advice. Although I have great respect for my consultant as both a surgeon and a person, the way he told me I had secondary cancer was very blunt. Both myself and my husband were left feeling traumatised, wondering how long I had left to live. As a 38 year old woman I felt as though my life was being stolen and the reduction in precious time I had with my husband filled me with panic. I was later reassured by a Macmillan nurse, who offered me the same information, but communicated it in a much more humane way. She was sensitive to my emotions, listened to my worries and consoled me without artificial sympathy. Why couldn't she have given me the news that I had secondaries in the first place?*
> **Pamela, breast cancer**

Being aware that the doctor may find it hard, too
It's often easy to forget that doctors and other health professionals aren't always very skilled at giving you the right information in the right amounts. If they have to give you bad news, or involve you in a difficult decision, that may also be a challenge for them. This doesn't mean that you have to be sorry for them or to put up with unhelpful behaviour, but it can be useful to remember that they might be struggling too.

> *It seems grossly unfair that every healthcare professional should have to think about, and monitor, not only what they say, but also the inference that can be placed on the words they use. However, I do think they should accept the responsibility and be prepared to learn the skills that will make communication easier, both for them and their patients.*

For a wide variety of reasons, patients may not have the ability to communicate with ease, which is not to say that they don't want to, or that they lack feelings. It is that category of patient who will be most reliant upon the healthcare professional to guide them through what may well be the worst experience in their life.

Karen, breast cancer

How health professionals respond to their patients is inevitably influenced by their experience of cancer in their personal lives. It is easy to forget that health professionals are also individuals – parents, partners, children, friends – as well as doctors, nurses etc. And unfortunately, the fact that they are health professionals doesn't make them immune from being affected by cancer in their own lives. However, you shouldn't have to feel that you are protecting them!

My thoughts are that [the doctor] *may have been as frightened of cancer as I was. We are about the same age and I may have been a mirror to his emotions. I wondered if his impatience with me was a fear of what might happen to him. His callous disregard of my position could be his discomfort with the condition he confronts with patients everyday. He diagnoses major cancers that are life threatening, leaving people months, or maybe weeks to live. After all mine was merely a little finger.*

Mark, sarcoma

Repeating back what you think you've heard, to check you've got it right
Misunderstandings frequently occur simply because of a different understanding of what has been said. It is useful to check back, using a phrase such as 'So what you are saying is . . . Have I got that right?' It is perfectly acceptable to ask for an explanation of anything you don't understand.

Privacy
It is difficult to feel at ease with your doctor or any other health professional if a conversation is taking place while you are having a physical examination, or you are waiting for an investigation or treatment while half undressed. While they may be used to it, that is no reason for you to accept it. Privacy and dignity are important for most people. Ask if you can get dressed first before continuing a conversation or request something to cover you up if you are still waiting to be seen.

At one of my periodic check ups, I was referred to an oncologist. His surgery was a bit shambolic the day I went, as his receptionist was unwell and he was trying to answer the door and so on. But he actually left me on the couch, naked to the waist to answer the 'phone. He left the door open and another patient passing the door could see me. This man gave me the impression he wasn't interested in what I wanted to ask, he wasn't interested in anything I had to say and even worse, he was very patronising. On the other hand, my surgeon's approach was very much to treat me as an adult and to answer my questions intelligently.

Anne, breast cancer

Talking to other members of the family

Think about who else you would like to be given information about you and tell your doctor what you want. You may find it helpful to ask your doctor to speak to other members of your family, especially if they have not been present at your appointment. Your doctor should be happy to talk to them with you there or separately, depending on your wishes.

After your appointment

Learning that you have a life threatening disease is more than likely to leave your head spinning with all kinds of thoughts that may be difficult to put into words. You may find it helpful to take some time before you go home to sit quietly and collect your thoughts. If you were not expecting to be told you have cancer you may not have thought to take anyone with you. Facing other people straight away can be quite daunting if you feel upset. Ask the doctor or nurse if there is somewhere you can sit for a few minutes. Some cancer centres and units have patient information and support centres where you can talk to someone who can support you and find information about other support services.

Shattering though it may be, the diagnosis may not be the only thing to cause anxiety at the first consultation. Although other worries may seem trivial on reflection, they can be very real at the time. Don't underestimate how everyday issues may make an already difficult situation harder to cope with. Transport and parking problems are perfect examples!

I had a biopsy because white spots had been found on my regular mammogram. In the literature sent to me about the clinic it gave information about the car park at the local supermarket which was free with a limit of two hours, and ten minutes walk from the hospital. I had to wait an hour to see the surgeon and then the consultation with him took about 45 minutes and then I had a half an hour with the nurse. From about half way into the session with the surgeon I was so anxious about whether my car would be clamped that I was thinking about that as much as what was being said about the biopsy results which were not good news (high grade DCIS [a type of breast cancer], with the need for a mastectomy [surgical removal of the breast]). I cried most of the way back to the car park as much in anxiety about my car and what I would do if it was clamped (I had neither my credit card nor cash with me) as I did about the bad news I had just received. If I had known it might take so long I would not have gone by car.

Ellen, breast cancer

Even if you were prepared for your diagnosis and had some questions thought through, you will now be trying to sort out the information the doctor has given you, to make some sense of it. Your thoughts may now be turning to how you tell your family and friends and what impact it will have on your life. Will you be able to continue working when you start treatment? What about the children? Perhaps you are already a carer and are worried about spending time in hospital. These questions will be explored more in depth in Chapter 4.

Resources

CancerBACUP

3 Bath Place, Rivington Street, London EC2A 3JR
Tel: 020 7696 9003 / Cancer Information Service: 0808 800 1234 (freephone)
www.cancerbacup.org.uk
Cancer nurses provide information and emotional support on all aspects of cancer. They produce a wide range of booklets and fact sheets on cancer, its treatments and the practical issues of coping including: Who can ever understand? – Talking about your cancer; Lost for words – How to talk to someone with cancer.

Macmillan Cancer Relief

89 Albert Embankment, London SE1 7UQ
Macmillan Cancerline: 0808 808 2020 (freephone)
www.macmillan.org.uk
Provides free information and support for people living with cancer. They also provide information on support groups throughout the country.

Useful reading

Cancer At Your Fingertips (2001) Val Speechley & Maxine Rosenfield.
Class Publishing, London. ISBN 1 85959 036 5

4
Sharing the diagnosis

Cancer turns lives upside down. After diagnosis, you will need both medical information about the cancer itself, and practical information to help you live with your cancer. Medical information will include information about symptoms, investigations, different treatment options and likely outcomes. Practical information can range from advice about the physical and emotional effects of having treatment through to coping with changes in family and social relationships, and work. You may also need information about administrative matters such as money, benefits, housing or employment rights.

What should you tell your family?

Just as it is hard when you first hear a diagnosis of cancer from the doctor, it is equally hard knowing how to tell family, friends and work colleagues. If you had someone with you at your appointment, you may find it helpful to discuss with them what was said. What your next step will be may depend on whether you need further investigations before treatment decisions can be made. It can be quite frustrating to be bombarded with questions that you can't answer until you have next seen your doctor. Equally, family and friends can be very supportive during this uncertain time and possibly suggest questions that you would like to ask on your next visit.

> *Telling my son who lives here was difficult enough. Telling my son and daughter who live in Canada was much more difficult. My son lives in Ontario and my daughter in Quebec. I felt so wrong giving them this bad news and not being there to reassure them. This I had to do twice.*
>
> *I was especially worried about my daughter. She was expecting her first child to arrive in January 1999 and he arrived in December 98, one month early. I'm sure my bad news had something to do with that although my daughter reassured me that it was just a coincidence. But I just couldn't put it out of my mind. Thanks heavens everything turned out to be OK.*
>
> **David, breast cancer**

Some people prefer to mull over the information they have been given, to come to terms with it themselves before telling anyone else. It is likely to depend on what your previous experience of cancer has been – if it has a negative, bad image or if you know people who have survived cancer.

I – we – struggled about what to tell my wider family. I had tried several things out on colleagues. One person I admired, I told I had bone cancer. That was all I knew then. She winced so alarmingly that I modified what I said to others. I became aware of the raw power of the word 'cancer'. Even doctors avoid using it. . . . My thoughts ran more along the lines of the effect that 'cancer' had on the faces of those I told. I realised that for some it means instant death and I saw revulsion in their eyes. For others it brings out huge sympathy. I began to respect it more and not to treat it so lightly. I asked my parents to let other family members know and that I would be happy to talk about it. Unfortunately, neither they nor others in my family asked anything. Such distance was already there and I should have known better than to suggest an open-minded approach. Except for one, a cousin who had been diagnosed with breast cancer some years ago and we were the only ones to speak to them. They heaped attention on me and it contributed to making me feeling rather special.

My immediate family were marvellous, my wife and our children. The silence from others was damning. I tried to dismiss it as 'typical of them', but secretly I had thought it would be different with me.

Mark, sarcoma

Families may have to adjust to the role changes that can result. For the breadwinner, to take on the care for children and running the home can seem daunting as well as tiring. And the partner who has been looking after the children and the house may need to work outside the home for the first time. It is not easy if you have to relinquish your role to others.

Talking with partners

For most people who are in stable relationships, the partner is likely to be the first line of support. If they were with you when you were given the news, they will have been able to share this news with you. Together, you will be able to go back over what was said and perhaps think of questions that you want to ask at your next appointment.

Maybe your partner was unable to accompany you to your appointment, or perhaps you were not expecting to need anyone with you. When a diagnosis of cancer comes out of the blue, there is no easy way to tell people close to you. It is not always possible to predict how another person will react to distressing news. While your reaction will be a reflection on how you cope best at the time, their reaction may also reflect how they are coping with the news. Just as you may feel angry at your diagnosis, your partner may also express feelings of anger at that time, and therefore may not seem particularly supportive. When we are hurt, we often take out our anger on other people. That does not mean to say that the anger is directed at any one individual, just that the nearest person tends to bear the brunt of it! Perhaps your partner seems remote and uninterested. It can be an extra burden, having to cope with another person's emotions at the same time as coping with your own. In the same way that your feelings will probably change over time, so will your partner's. His or her life will be just as affected by the diagnosis as yours will be.

Not all partners end up being much help and single parents, in particular, sometimes find support is not forthcoming. Sadie, whose former partner no longer lives with the family, needed to tell him of her likely diagnosis because of the impact her treatment would have on their children.

I made the mistake, after I'd seen the physician the first time and I'd had the barium enema, I wrote to my former partner, who lives in the same area. I didn't want to speak to him on the telephone because of the children. I wrote to him and said, 'I'm going to have to have an operation, I think the likelihood is I've got cancer and I'm going to need you to have the children to stay and I'm going to need some extra money because someone is going to have to look after these children. I know that the childminder, a nanny that comes in, would come daily but she's going to have to stay, I'm going to have to pay her a lot more and I'm going to need some help'. He telephoned and as his mother had bowel [colon] cancer the previous year, he said well 'How far is this cancer advanced, ask them about the staging'. I'd never heard of staging. I said 'I don't know what you're talking about' and he then said, 'Oh well, if you've got a D stage, there's no hope, it's terminal'. I didn't really want to hear this at that moment, as it was not helpful information to have at that time. I'll draw a veil over him because he didn't come up with the extra money and when I had to stay in hospital after three weeks, he also didn't turn up to take the children at the weekend. They were left one evening sitting there with their suitcases packed and my eldest daughter and the nanny had to try and sort it all out. He just phoned and said he was not coming, because I'd also had arranged with him to have them for three weekends. He said, 'Why three, you'll be out after two' and I told him I thought I might feel a bit tired.

Sadie, colon cancer

What about people who don't have a partner, or a family member they are close to or who lives nearby? Often it can be friends who make up the support network. Even when there is family support, some people feel they would prefer the support of a close friend.

I had taken the day off work to go to my god-daughter's christening. I went to my GP in the morning as I'd made an appointment to find out the result of my second mammogram. I got home and I can remember sitting there and thinking I couldn't move. It was about three o'clock because I had intended to catch the 1.30 train from Waterloo and I think my friend was going to pick me up half past four. She was going to pick me up and in the end, I arrived at 9.15 or something like that. And she was getting really worried by then, she was 'phoning everybody she knew because by then I should have been there. And I remember that in the car, I told her what happened and I was trying not to cry. I remember that, and I remember her saying to me, 'What do you want me to do, do you want me to tell every one', because it was the christening that weekend. Her family were going to be there and lots of friends were coming. When I arrived her two brothers were already there, waiting for me to have supper and I said don't tell anyone, I just wanted you to know. The whole weekend it was like I went through this process of being there and not being there. But looking back, in some ways it was a very good thing I was among so many people because I really don't know how I would have coped, had I been completely on my own.

Dee, breast cancer

Telling the children

Telling children, particularly young children, is never going to be easy. So much will depend on your relationship with them and how you may have dealt with other crises in the past. The family is always affected and children are sensitive to change, especially when it threatens the future of the family. But the experience of many parents with cancer who have been faced with this situation, suggests it is usually best to be honest. This doesn't mean you necessarily want to give your children every piece of information you have. How much information, and when, will obviously depend on the age and emotional maturity of the children.

I had to tell my children (aged 5 to 15 years) and I had to decide what I was going to tell them. I'm really ashamed to say that I had decided I would give them more and more information, bit by bit. But I decided I wasn't going to tell them that I had cancer because cancer in our family had a very negative, bad image as three out of their four grandparents had died with cancer. So I had to find a way of reframing cancer positively and feel comfortable with it myself before I could give the information to them. I think you're in a difficult position when you don't have all the information yourself but you've still got to give it to other people. I told them what I could and, in the end, I did tell them I had cancer.

Sadie, colon cancer

Honesty means acknowledging to your children that you have an illness, and that the doctors are going to give you treatment to make you better. If you know that the treatment may make you feel worse for a time, tell them. Maintaining secrecy around the diagnosis can be very stressful and isolating. You will probably have to repeat the information you give them and frequently check their understanding. Give them time to come to terms with the information and an opportunity to ask questions. Ask them if they have heard any words that they don't understand or find frightening. Allow them to express how they are feeling and reassure them that they are loved.

One major decision was what to tell my daughter, who was then only ten. We have always been very close and communicate openly on everything, so I decided to be truthful. Obviously I had to frame the facts in a way that was as comprehensible and non-threatening as possible, but it's worked out well for us. Being honest with her means that she trusts me completely and never has concerns that I'm hiding unpalatable news.

Karen, breast cancer

Younger children in particular require reassurance that it is nothing they have said or done that has caused this situation. Children invariably know that something is wrong and trying to protect them by not saying anything may lead them to imagine far worse scenarios. Tom and Jane decided not to tell their children aged eight and eleven years that their father had cancer until the treatment or disease started causing obvious problems. Not unnaturally, they didn't want to cause them any unnecessary distress or worry. The downside to this was the parents decided not to confide in close family or friends for fear that the children might overhear about the diagnosis from someone else. When they did eventually to talk to the children and could then be open with the rest of the family, they likened it to 'an umbrella of support opening up'. Telling the children was an emotional time and they were as worried about becoming too upset themselves as they were about their children's reactions. However, this opened up opportunities for the children to ask questions about the disease and to express their feelings about it. Looking back, Tom and Jane wished that they had talked as a family earlier.

You may find telling your children yourselves too painful, and prefer to ask a close family member or a trusted friend to take on this role. It is very important for children to be given an explanation for the disruption within the family and the chance to explore feelings and ask questions. Children will need reassurance that they can't 'catch' cancer. They will also need reassurance that they were in no way responsible for you developing it.

Some children may not seem to be affected in any way. This doesn't mean that they don't feel anything, just that their way of coping is to shut it out. Let them know that they can talk about how they feel at any time, and that you will try and answer any questions as best you can.

If you are part of a family that is not used to crying in front of each other, you may find an emotional conversation difficult to cope with. Choose a time that feels right for you. On the other hand, crying together as a family gives children the message that it is OK to cry. By sharing information with them, you can offer them support.

There are bound to be disruptions to family life when a parent is ill and it will not always be possible for family life to continue normally. Depending on the ages of the children, some aspects of normality (such as attending school) will need to continue. In families where the only parent has cancer, this can place additional responsibilities on the older children – caring for younger children, cooking and other household tasks. It is important for all children, whatever their age, to have some time to themselves, to be with friends where they can continue to enjoy their own interests and have fun.

I asked to see the social worker at the hospital. As my stay in hospital went on and on, my needs for childcare did not diminish. It started to get quite anxiety provoking. I asked if I could have, just for a couple of weeks, some sort of home help. I was very clear what I needed and it was very minimal. A couple of hours a week for three or four weeks to help me actually do the things I had to do, to look after my family. But they couldn't provide that because they provide personal care. I couldn't do things like making beds or prepare meals and they expected, I think unfairly, my oldest children to do it all. What they really needed after the experience they'd been through was for someone to look after them. What they did not need – they were only fifteen and thirteen – was to have to look after me and cook all their own meals and all that sort of thing. They needed to be able to play.

Sadie, colon cancer

Older children may have different or additional problems. The teenage years can be hard enough in any circumstances without having to cope with a parent who is ill.

Depending on how your child is coping at school, you may feel it helpful to tell the teachers. Sometimes, stress or worry can result in behaviour changes, with the child becoming either withdrawn or disruptive. Teachers who know what is behind such changes will be in a better position to offer help and support. Some children find it comforting to tell close friends what is happening, others may prefer not to. Individual choices about who to tell and when should be respected just as thoroughly in children as in adults.

Telling a parent

Just as sharing your diagnosis with children can be painful, it can also be hard to tell a parent. Most parents envisage dying before their children – it's the natural way. To be told that a child – even an adult child – has a life threatening diagnosis is going to be difficult for a parent, whatever their age. So if your parents are themselves frail or unwell, you may feel it is unhelpful to tell them. How often you see them and the type of relationship you have with them will also be factors affecting when and what you tell. While attitudes are changing, older people may still be uncomfortable talking about cancer.

When I was first diagnosed in 1991, cancer wasn't spoken about as much as it was when I developed my second primary four years later. It was still a dirty word and it never occurred to me to question it. My mother was very shocked when I spoke about it openly and I noticed that people of her generation actually crossed the street, rather than speak to me. In 1995 people were speaking about it much more openly.

Anne, breast cancer

I'd been backwards and forwards to hospital for numerous investigations, so I don't think my father was overly surprised when I said that I had something important to tell him. I had to mute the television in order to get his attention, after which he looked everywhere but at me and said not a word. Before I'd left the room, the television volume was turned up again. I understood that he couldn't find the words to respond to my news, but the complete lack of response was very distressing.

Karen, breast cancer

Telling friends

The decision to discuss your diagnosis with friends is yours alone. However, it is usually best to be honest about your cancer with people close to you. Keeping it a secret can cause you more stress at a time when you could use the support of others. Remember, too, that your friends will probably learn about your cancer at some point. If and when they do, they may feel hurt and left out if you haven't told them, which may make it harder for them to be supportive.

Many people say that having a life threatening disease has changed their lives in countless ways. This extends to friendships. Which friends to tell and when, will often be influenced by the reaction you expect from them. However, you may want some time to think through what you are going to say, when you are going to say it, and to whom.

I had a certain amount of information, as much as I could cope with at that time. I had to leave it for a few days and come to terms with it myself before I started telling anybody else. I had to start feeling comfortable and confidant and positive about it myself before I could tell other people. All my friends were just so marvellous because I just found a way of saying to them all 'I've got cancer and we're going to be very positive about this and it's not the end of the world'. You could see immediately the moment you said you've got cancer, you could see in their faces that they were going to say how dreadful and I'd immediately say but I'm feeling very positive. They would all take their cue from me, they were just so supportive.

Sadie, colon cancer

Sometimes friendships fall by the wayside, as people can't cope with the new situation. Equally, friends or acquaintances who may have been on the perimeter of a social circle, can come to the fore in a surprising way. While you are not responsible for their reactions and emotions, you may sometimes feel that it is you supporting them rather than the other way round!

Dealing with other people's reactions is difficult. Compassion fatigue sets in very quickly, even with the closest of friends, so you learn to put a brave face on things. It's an obvious relief to most people that you don't moan about your problems, but it can be upsetting that they appear so eager to take things at face value, and don't seem to realise that you're trying to spare them!

Karen, breast cancer

Quite often during my illness I felt I needed to be strong for other people and protect them from my diagnosis of cancer rather than it being the other way round. It was like making believe I was coping with it all really well instead of being at death's door. Other people's anxieties were sometimes harder to deal with than my own. In my case, I never doubted my own recovery but because people always associate cancer with death it takes patience to show people otherwise.

Nina, sarcoma

It can often be helpful to let family and friends know how they can best support you. They may not know whether or not you want to talk about your diagnosis. Or they might not know enough about cancer to have any understanding of what you are going through. It is often through providing you with practical help that people can really show their support. If you are feeling more tired than usual, the most helpful thing could be for someone to take over some of your shopping or housework, particularly if you live on your own. Not everyone wants or needs practical help, however, and you should feel able to decline offers of help if they are not appropriate.

The telephone never stops, if you've got somebody in the family ill in hospital. You get sick to death of telling the story. You soon learn which people drain you of your vitality, the people who are 'phoning you for comfort. But even the ones you want to speak to, that you know love you and you know care about you, you get physically worn out telling the same story over and over again, particularly if it's an upsetting story and you know you're going to upset them. Some days you feel able to talk about it. What I did was organise a sort of, like a relay, I'd 'phone one friend and she'd 'phone another one.

Anne, breast cancer

Telling work colleagues

Cancer impacts on an individual's identity in the workplace and can threaten job and financial security. You will need to tell your employer that you are likely to require time off to attend hospital appointments. Many employers are very supportive and by having an understanding attitude can take some of the stress out of the situation, allowing individuals to focus their energies on getting well. Unfortunately, this will not always be the case, particularly for people who have been in a job for a relatively short time. Your employer or personnel officer will be able to give you guidance on how much time you can take off for medical appointments and how much sick leave you are entitled to while undergoing treatment. Some larger organisations provide occupational health services for their employees, where you discuss your situation in confidence.

It is important to keep employers informed about your situation, as this will help them to support you and plan cover for any absences. However, not all employers are able to offer support if prolonged absence affects their business – which it certainly will do after a relatively short time if the organisation you work for is small. Many people may go through a period when their financial situation causes them great stress. This worry can be even greater for people who are self-employed as they may fear no one will want to put work their way again. The Department of Work and Pensions can give you advice on benefits and information on employment rights. While no one can be dismissed purely for having cancer, an employer can dismiss a person who is unable to carry out his or her job because of illness. If you are worried your job may be at risk, you may find it helpful to talk to Citizens Advice (www.citizensadvice.org.uk) or local legal advice centre.

I had just started a new job for a small health charity (who received funds from the government (DFID) for Third World Health projects ironically) when my early cancer symptoms were becoming more noticeable. At the time, I was on a probationary period and unaware of my illness – I just knew I was tired all the time and didn't know why. I put it down to my long commute, the stresses of a new job, personal worries and even bugs from a trip overseas causing me to feel constantly run down. I decided I needed to seek more medical advice to find out why I was feeling so bad. My new employers were now not happy with my constant medical visits. They were more annoyed than concerned even after I found a lump near my knee and was visibly limping around the office in pain for three weeks. I was finally rushed into hospital via emergency after much misdiagnosis.

> *My employers never treated me like I had a legitimate concern about an illness in the period leading up to my cancer diagnosis. Until you are actually in treatment the early symptoms of cancer are often confusing for everyone. In my experience, I was instead treated like a bad employee – after all I was tired all the time. It was even more disappointing to find out that when I was finally diagnosed with a sarcoma and it became clear I would need long term treatment and chemotherapy – they would terminate my contract. I was on a probationary period and they were within their rights to do so.*
>
> **Nina, sarcoma**

Your immediate colleagues may also be good friends, but this is not always the case. However, they are the ones most likely to notice if you are having to take a lot of time off. Having said this, the decision who to tell and when to tell should be yours. Just because you tell your boss that you might need time off, this doesn't mean that you have to tell all your work colleagues.

As the effects of cancer treatment vary from person to person, it is not always easy to anticipate in advance how you will cope. The type of treatment you have will obviously make a difference to how it will affect your job. You may find that treatment interferes surprisingly little with your ability to continue working or you may find that you have to make adjustments. To a large extent, it will depend on the type of work you do. If you do develop financial problems as a result of being unable to work or perhaps need help with the cost of child-care, you can find information on benefits and other services through your local benefits agency or hospital social work team.

Resources

CancerBACUP
3 Bath Place, Rivington Street, London EC2A 3JR
Tel: 020 7696 9003 / Cancer Information Service: 0808 800 1234 (freephone)
www.cancerbacup.org.uk
Cancer nurses provide information and emotional support on all aspects of cancer.
They produce a wide range of booklets and fact sheets on cancer, its treatments and the practical issues of coping including: Sexuality and Cancer

Department of Work and Pensions
Olympic House, Olympic Way, Wembley, Middlesex HA9 0DL
Helpline 0800 88 22 00
www.dwp.gov.uk
Gives advice on benefits and information on employment rights.

Institute of Family Therapy
24–32 Stephenson Way, London NW1 2HX
Tel: 020 7391 9150
www.instituteoffamilytherapy.org.uk
Offers counselling for families, including those in which a family member has a serious illness or where there has been a bereavement.

Cancerlink at Macmillan Cancer Relief
89 Albert Embankment, London SE1 7UQ
Macmillan Cancerline: 0808 808 2020 (freephone)
www.macmillan.org.uk
Produces a range of publications about day to day practical and emotional issues including: Talking to children when an adult has cancer.

Child Bereavement Trust
Aston House, High Street, West Wycombe, Bucks HP14 3AG
Tel: 01494 446 648
www.childbereavement.org.uk
They provide resources and information for bereaved children, families and health professionals including the booklet: When Your Mum or Dad has Cancer, *for children who have a seriously ill parent.*

National Association of Citizens Advice Bureaux (NACAB)
115–123 Pentonville Road, London N1 9LZ
Tel: 020 7833 2181
www.citizensadvice.org.uk
Can provide a list of local Citizens Advice Bureaux.

Relate
Herbert Gray College, Little Church Street, Rugby, Warwickshire CV21 3AP
Tel: 0845 4561310 *or* 01788 573241
www.relate.org.uk
Offers relationship counselling via local branches. They also have RELATELINE *(helpline: 0845 130 40 10) if you want to talk to someone right now. Relateline gives you the opportunity to ask questions and can offer ideas and direction for the future. It operates from 9.30am to 4.30pm, Monday to Friday and calls are charged at local rates. All calls are entirely confidential.*

Useful reading

Challenging Cancer (2002), by Maurice Slevin & Nira Kfir, Class Publishing, London. ISBN 1 85959 068 3. See the chapters on 'Family relationships: discussion with supporters', and 'Talking with children'.

5
Making choices
about treatment

Many people want to know as much as possible about their cancer, the different types of treatment available to them, and any potential side effects. This information helps some people to make some sort of sense of their illness. When treatment can last for weeks or months, having information at the beginning can help you to plan your life around it. Information can also help you to cope more effectively with potential side effects. Even though you may want information, this doesn't necessarily mean that you always want to take part in making decisions about your treatment. However, having a choice about whether to take part in making decisions can help you to feel more in control.

Not everyone wants detailed information about their cancer and its treatment, and if this is the right option for you your choices should be respected. It should be up to you to decide how much information you want and how involved you wish to be in making decisions. Doctors are not mind readers, so make sure you tell your doctor. You may find that over time you want more information. This is a normal reaction but, again, your doctors will not know it is happening to you unless you tell them.

When treatment options are being discussed, it's very easy to misinterpret what's being said. Healthcare professionals deal with these issues on a daily basis and can sound much too laid back about possible side effects and outcome of treatments. Sometimes it would be easy to believe that they see you as a disease on legs and have lost sight of just how personal the issues are to you. We're all far too well behaved to say, 'For goodness sake, why are you being so casual when it's my life on the line?' but perhaps we sometimes should! Extracting information can be akin to getting blood from a stone. After a long wait you get into the consulting room and what you really want to get out of the way first are the results of your investigations. The last thing you want is to sit eye to eye with the doctor, wondering why he, or she, is so reluctant to tell you what's afoot. Are they trying to avoid a difficult issue, or is it a control thing? It can sometimes turn into a cat and mouse game of who's going to cave in first and refer to the results of the dreaded tests!

Karen, breast cancer

While this book hasn't been written to provide you with information about the different treatment options available, it may be helpful to provide a brief overview of the most common treatments.

- **Surgery** is a common treatment which aims to remove all or as much of the tumour as possible. It is a *local* treatment (i.e. a treatment of a very specific part of the body), and is still the first treatment of choice in curing many cancers.

- **Radiotherapy** is the use of high energy rays to damage cancer cells and stop them dividing. It is sometimes called radiation therapy. Radiation is used in medicine both for diagnosis and investigation (x-rays), and for treatment (radiotherapy). Even though radiation can be dangerous, when it is used properly the benefits greatly outweigh the risks. Radiotherapy may be used on its own to treat cancer, or in conjunction with other treatments such as surgery and/or chemotherapy. It is a *localised* treatment as it only destroys cells in the area of the body being treated. Treatment can either be given from outside the body (external radiotherapy), or from within (internal radiotherapy), by placing radioactive treatment material in or close to the tumour being treated.

- **Chemotherapy** is treatment with cytotoxic drugs to destroy cancer cells (*cyto* means 'cell', *toxic* means 'poisonous'). It can be referred to as a *systemic* therapy, as the drugs are carried around the whole body (the 'system') in the bloodstream and destroy the cancer cells by damaging their ability to reproduce. Sometimes one drug is used or it may be a combination of several drugs, taken from a selection of about 40 different drugs available. Chemotherapy may be used alone to treat cancer or in conjunction with other treatments such as surgery and/or radiotherapy.

- **Hormone therapy** (endocrine treatment) can be a treatment option for certain cancers. When a tumour occurs in a part of the body (such as the ovary or prostate) that depends on hormones for its functions, the tumour can also be dependent on hormones. In these cancers, treatment involves blocking hormones, stopping their production or changing the way they work. Hormone therapy is usually taken by mouth (orally) and sometimes can be given in a course of injections. The best known example at present is Tamoxifen, which is used in the treatment of breast cancer.

- **Bone marrow and peripheral blood stem cell transplants** may be used for certain cancers. These include some leukaemias, lymphomas or breast cancer, where treatment with high doses of chemotherapy and/or radiotherapy offers an increased chance of cure. The effect of treatment can depress the bone marrow and delay recovery, and bone marrow and stem cell transplants can help speed up the recovery process. The bone marrow or stem cells are removed or 'harvested' from you before the high dose treatment is given, stored, and then returned to you by a vein like a blood transfusion.

- **Biological therapy** (also called **immunotherapy**) is treatment to stimulate the body's immune system to fight infection and disease. It is still in the experimental stages and is not yet part of standard treatment. Research is currently being carried out into the possible development of 'designer drugs' to target specific proteins that are important for the survival and growth of tumours.

- **Cancer vaccines (gene therapies)** are used in specific cancers such as malignant melanoma, prostate and colon cancers, to stimulate the immune system to produce its own antibodies to the cancer cells (in the same way as vaccinations against polio, for example). These treatments are still at an experimental stage and are therefore available in a few centres only.

Not all treatments will be suitable for each type of cancer. Treatment recommendations take into account the type of cancer, the stage of the disease, your individual medical history and your own preferences.

'Getting the best from your cancer services: Questions for Patients to Ask'

This report from the Commission for Health Improvement (CHI) and the Audit Commission was mentioned in Chapter 2 (see pages 27–8).

The questions displayed on the page opposite have been taken from the leaflet and are ones you may wish to ask when you are discussing treatment and care.

- How quickly will the treatment start?

- What will the treatment be like and how long will it take? Will there be side effects and what can I do about them?

- Is my surgeon a specialist in my form of cancer? Is this important for my type of cancer?

- Is the doctor prescribing my chemotherapy an oncologist? Will the nurses on hand during the chemotherapy have the right training?

- Can I have the chemotherapy in my local hospital?

- Can my surgery, radiotherapy or chemotherapy be speeded up by being performed outside normal office hours?

- Will my treatment be discussed by a multidisciplinary team? Does this team include cancer nurses as well as doctors?

- Will all the hospitals I attend know about my diagnosis and treatment?

- Who should I contact if I am worried about my diagnosis, treatment or prognosis?

- What help is available for my family? What patient support groups are there in my area?

- Will I need special equipment or support when I go home? Will I get this? Does my GP know I am being discharged?

- Who should I contact if I have questions or concerns, once my treatment has finished?

- What are the guidelines and standards for my treatment and care? Can I see them?

Informed consent

What is consent? Health professionals must have your consent or permission before they carry out any form of examination or treatment. You have a choice as to whether you say yes or no. But having this choice depends on your having enough information about the risks, as well as the benefits, of the treatment or investigation that is being offered to you. Before you make up your mind, you may want to ask for more information – or have it explained in a different way if you don't understand. Even after you have signed a consent form, you are free to change your mind at any stage without affecting your future care.

> *When I was first diagnosed with breast cancer, I signed the consent form for a lumpectomy. My surgeon was absolutely adamant that a mastectomy* [surgical removal of the breast] *wasn't appropriate or necessary because the tumour was so close to the chest wall. I would be left with a fairly decent shaped breast. When I came round from the lumpectomy my surgeon told me he had found a second primary site which he hadn't removed at the biopsy because it was in another part of the breast. He took away much more than he and I imagined he would and I asked him if another site was a cause for concern. He said it was and it was unexpected and didn't show up on the x-ray and then I asked him did he regret that he hadn't done a mastectomy because it was crossed off the consent form. After a lot of thought, he said no, the radiotherapy would take care of it. I did wonder whether I'd had the right treatment but I trusted him and he'd given it a lot of thought.*
>
> *The breast care nurse told me afterwards at the second diagnosis, four years later, that in the beginning, I was offered a choice of mastectomy and no further treatment or a lumpectomy and radiotherapy and I've no memory of that. I absolutely have no memory of that. All I remember is the surgeon saying we only want to do the minimum surgery. I've no memory of being offered a mastectomy and I would have definitely not chosen it. I coped as well as I did when I was first diagnosed because I felt that I still had a breast.*
>
> **Anne, breast cancer**

There are different ways in which you can give your consent. This could be simply offering up your arm when a nurse asks to take your blood pressure. By offering your arm you are giving consent without actually saying anything in words. Sometimes you will give your spoken consent, and at other times in writing by signing a form. The main conditions that ensure your consent is valid are: that you must be competent to make a decision, that you have received enough information to make that decision and that you are acting of your own free will. Having information isn't much help if you don't understand it. The whole concept of informed consent rests upon your having been given enough information by health professionals, using language that you can understand, for you to make up your mind about the best course of action for you. As well as the opportunity to discuss your treatment with your doctors, you can expect to be given written information to back up what you've been told. Different people want different amounts of information. You may want to know as much as possible about your cancer and possible treatments. On the other hand, you may prefer to leave the decisions to the health professionals.

When I went back to see the surgeon a week after I was diagnosed, he said he'd like me to see an oncologist to 'discuss treatments and tests and things'. This was my first glimmer of hope. I went to see her and from then on all my tests and everything were taken over by another hospital. I was quite happy there because I felt I'd had time all the way through the talks to decide what I wanted to do. I was consulted all the way through. I was more or less in control of what was going to happen and, rightly or wrongly, I wasn't pressed into doing one thing or the other.

Matthew, bladder *cancer*

When you are first diagnosed, you may well feel overwhelmed by the amount of information you are being asked to take in. Yet you are being asked to agree to treatments that may, for a time, make you feel worse than the actual disease. This will be particularly true if your cancer has been diagnosed early, before symptoms have become troublesome. Having information in small chunks can be one way of keeping on top of the situation. As you become more familiar with what is happening to you, you will probably find your information needs do change. It is important to remember that you are the one who can control the amount of information you are given. You can always ask for more information at any time. Some people find that it isn't until their treatment has finished that they feel ready to deal with what has been happening to them.

In order to make a decision about treatment, you will need two kinds of information. First of all, the health professionals need to discuss with you the medical details about the treatment such as the benefits, risks and side effects – information that you can't necessarily be expected to know. Then there is the information that relates to you as an individual. How will you personally be affected by the treatment, how will it affect your lifestyle and individual circumstances? What is important to one person may be less important to another, depending on your lifestyle, culture and background. This is a two way process and as well as giving you information, health professionals must listen to your questions and answer them as best they can.

One thing I decided very early on was that I wasn't going to lose my hair. I'd had friends who'd had treatment with chemotherapy who'd lost their hair. My information was very out of date then. I'd got a friend who's had leukaemia she had radical chemotherapy of course and we'd seen her lose her hair. I do listen a lot to the radio in the weekends and I used regularly to listen to the programme Medicine Now and I'd heard about cold cap therapy. I thought I'm not going to lose my hair, I don't have to lose my hair. One of the first things I asked when they said I had to have chemo was 'Do you have cold cap therapy' and it was only then that they said yes, but you won't need it because you won't lose your hair.

Sadie, colon cancer

There is a fine line between providing enough information to make an informed decision and listening to the wishes of individuals. The guidance from the General Medical Council (GMC) recommends that doctors should provide the following information:

- The purpose of the investigation or treatment;

- Details and uncertainties of the diagnosis;

- Options for treatment including the option not to treat;

- Explanation of the likely benefits and probabilities of success for each option;

- Known possible side effects;

- The name of the doctor who will have overall responsibility; and

- A reminder that you, the patient, can change your mind at any time.

Even when you don't wish to be involved in making decisions, doctors must still provide basic information about the treatment before proceeding.

There have been problems in the past about the process by which patients and relatives can give informed consent. To manage these problems, the Department of Health has introduced further consent forms. These help NHS organisations to improve the way patients are asked to give consent for treatment, care or research. One of the main features of these new consent forms is that they will document the key benefits and risks associated with the proposed procedure, and any additional information given to the patient. A copy of the page documenting the details of the treatment is offered to the patient.

To help you think about what you want to ask your doctor, you may find the following questions helpful. These have been taken from an information leaflet *About the consent form* which accompanies the Department of Health publication *Good practice in consent implementation guide: consent to examination or treatment*. This document, which is a guide for health professionals, was published in 2001. They are included here, however, to give you an idea of what your doctor's agenda might be before you frame your questions for him or her.

Questions may be about the **treatment itself**, for example:

- What are the main treatment options?

- What are the benefits of each of the options?

- What are the risks, if any, of each option?

- What are the success rates for different options – nationally, for this unit or for you (the surgeon)?

- Why do you think an operation (if suggested) is necessary?

- What are the risks if I decide to do nothing for the time being?

- How can I expect to feel after the procedure?

- When am I likely to be able to get back to work?

Questions may also be about how the treatment might affect your future state of health or style of life, for example:

- Will I need long-term care?

- Will my mobility be affected?

- Will I still be able to drive?

- Will it affect the kind of work I do?

- Will it affect my personal/sexual relationships?

- Will I be able to take part in my favourite sport/exercises?

- Will I be able to follow my usual diet?

The Department of Health publishes five guides to consent. You can find the details of these booklets through the DoH website www.doh.gov.uk/consent or you can obtain copies through the post by telephone or writing to them (see page 151). Copies may also be available through your local information centre.

Consent – What you have a right to expect:

- A guide for adults
- A guide for children and young people
- A guide for people with learning difficulties
- A guide for parents
- A guide for relatives and parents

Ask your doctor how long you can take to think through your decision. It will not necessarily be easy to weigh up all the positive and negative aspects of any proposed treatment. Many people worry that they need to decide immediately they have been diagnosed. This is not necessarily the case. Often these beliefs come about from the emphasis that is put on the importance of early diagnosis and treatment being essential to good outcomes. It helps to remember that different cancers behave in different ways – and some cancers grow much faster than others. While it may be important to start treatment as soon as possible, many people will have plenty of time to think about the various options. Ask any questions you think will help you to make a decision. Equally important, if you don't want to hear something you must make this clear to your doctor.

Here are some additional questions you may want to ask your consultant or specialist:

- How many people do you see with my type of cancer?
- What are the different treatment options available to me?
- How long can I take to decide about what treatment I have?
- Will these treatments cure me?
- When will I know if they have worked?
- Will I have to spend any time in hospital?
- How often will I need treatment?
- How long will my treatment go on for?
- How will I feel during treatment and are there any side effects I can expect?
- If there are any side effects, what can be done to help me cope with them?
- How long will it take for me to recover after I have finished the treatment?

- Are there any long-term side effects?
- Will I be able to continue with the same lifestyle that I'm leading now?
- What will happen if this treatment doesn't work?
- Can I talk to someone who has had the same treatment?
- Who else can I talk to about my cancer?
- Are my children more at risk of developing a cancer because I have cancer?
- Will I be able to have a family after the treatment? (if applicable)
- Do I have to be in a clinical trial to have this treatment? (if applicable)

Clinical trials

You may be invited to take part in a clinical trial or other research study to help find new or improved treatments for cancer, especially if you are receiving treatment in a specialist centre.

Separate consent is always sought for research studies and you should be given sufficient information to allow you to decide whether or not you want to take part. When a new treatment is thought to offer benefits over the best-known standard treatment, comparisons of the two are made within the setting of a clinical trial. This may involve comparing drugs, radiotherapy or different operations. The effectiveness of the new treatment and any possible side effects have to be assessed before it can be widely used for all people with a particular cancer.

The NHS Cancer Research Network (NCRN)

The NHS Cancer Research Network (NCRN) is being developed to co-ordinate cancer research across the country. It is a key part of the National Cancer Research Institute (NCRI), which is a partnership between government, the voluntary sector and the private sector. The institute will identify the areas where research is most needed and likely to improve areas of treatment, diagnosis and care. The Cancer Research Network, which will mirror the cancer services networks, aims to increase the number of adults entering cancer trials. This should lead to better quality clinical research and make sure that the research evidence will be incorporated into cancer care.

Types of clinical trials

Randomised trial

Randomised trials compare different treatments and patients may receive the new treatment or the best-known standard treatment. A computer selects the treatment for each individual, not the doctors.

Double blind trial

In a double blind trial, neither you nor your doctor will know which treatment group you are in. However, if your doctor needs to find out this information, it will be possible to do so.

Placebo

A placebo is an inactive substance for example, in the form of a pill which looks like the real thing but is not. It contains no active ingredient.

Phase I studies

Phase I studies find out what is the most effective dose of a treatment, and the side effects of the drug.

Phase II studies

Phase II studies build on Phase I studies. They look at the dose and frequency of treatment, and which cancers may respond best.

Phase III studies

In Phase III studies, a new treatment is compared with the best-known standard treatment.

Clinical drug trials are only set up once a drug has been shown to be both safe and effective in laboratory and animal studies. All clinical trials have to be approved by a research ethics committee, made up of doctors and other non-medical people. They will decide whether the potential benefits outweigh the possible risks.

The researcher will explain the trial to you and give you a written information sheet. Many doctors have research nurses working with them who can also answer your questions and provide support throughout the trial. If you decide that you wish to take part in the study you will be asked to give your verbal or written consent. You can withdraw from a trial at any time without affecting your overall treatment and care. If the particular treatment being used does not benefit you then the doctors will discuss alternative treatment with you.

Clinical trials are not always explained well. True, you get told about the basic remit, but that isn't always enough. I was invited to join a clinical trial, which would have been a lifeline to me. At the last moment the offer was withdrawn, because I failed to meet all the clinical criteria for the trial, which allowed for no flexibility. There had been no information given about the criteria that had to be satisfied and there was no explanation as to why this hadn't been checked earlier. No apology was forthcoming about dashing my hopes, nor did anyone seem to recognise how upset I felt.

Karen, breast cancer

During a research study, you will be closely observed and data on your case will be carefully recorded to monitor your progress. This data will be kept confidential. If you agree to take part in any trial, the research nurse involved in your study will explain any extra visits, blood tests or investigations that are necessary. Here are some of the questions you may wish to ask if you are considering taking part in a clinical trial.

- What is the purpose of this study?

- Why have I been chosen?

- Do I have to take part?

- What will happen to me if I take part?

- What do I have to do?

- What is the drug or procedure that is being tested?

- How long will the study last?

- How could the trial help me?

- What are the side effects of taking part?

- What are the benefits and risks?

- Will I need any extra tests or investigations?

- What other treatments are available if I don't take part in this trial?

- Who can I contact if I have any concerns or problems?

- What if new information becomes available?

- What happens when the research study stops?

- What if something goes wrong?

- Will my taking part in this study be kept confidential?

- What will happen to the results of the research study?

- Who is organising and funding the research?

(Source: Department of Health (2001) *Consent – what you have a right to expect: A guide for adults*)

National Cancer Improving Outcomes Guidance

A group of health experts has produced guidance documents for specific cancer types to help NHS Trusts to review and develop their cancer services. These documents look at how cancer services should be organised in order to provide the best treatment and care to ensure the best outcomes. For each cancer site, a group of experts – professionals, people with personal experience of the cancer and academics – pooled their experience and knowledge of the disease. They came up with proposals for recommendations that were sent to a wide range of people for comment. The resulting documents include practical guidance for developing services and a review of the supporting research evidence.

To date, guidance has been produced on the following cancer types:

- *Breast cancer* (1996) – the original guidance has been updated by NICE (see opposite) for the NHS in England and Wales and is called *Improving Outcomes in Breast Cancer: Update*. They have updated some of the original recommendations, added further recommendations and have also produced information for the public.
- Colorectal [bowel] cancer (1997)
- Lung cancer (1998)
- Gynaecological [women's] cancer (1999)
- Upper gastrointestinal [stomach, throat, oesophagus] cancers (2002)
- Urological [prostate, testicular, penile, bladder, kidney] cancers (2002)

Other cancer service guidance is in progress.

The NHS Prostate Cancer Programme (2000) looks at prostate cancer screening and the research needed to improve cancer services for men with prostate cancer.

These documents are available through the Department of Health website www.doh.gov.uk/cancer or you can obtain a copy by writing to the Department at the address given on page 151.

The National Institute for Clinical Excellence (NICE)

High quality treatment and care should be available to everyone with cancer, regardless of where in the country they live. However, there are variations in the quality of care and treatment across the country. To ensure fairer access to the most effective treatments, NICE was set up by the government in 1999. Its role is to provide patients, health professionals and the public with guidance on current 'best practice' in medicine (including cancer) in England and Wales. NICE reviews existing treatments and assesses new treatments for cost-effectiveness as well as other benefits. This will help overcome the 'postcode lottery' (i.e. having the quality of your treatment determined by where you happen to live).

In addition to publishing guidance on new cancer drugs, NICE is carrying out a comprehensive review of the organisation of cancer services.

The NICE guidance *Improving Outcomes in Breast Cancer: Manual Update* is the first document to be published by the institute in a series of site-specific (for example, breast, lung) cancer guidelines which aims to support the NHS. Their website www.nice.org.uk provides further details about other cancer guidelines coming out in the future.

Can I refuse treatment?

You are entitled to refuse treatment if you are a competent adult, even if this results in permanent physical injury or your death. All treatments carry risks as well as benefits. How risks are weighed up will vary enormously between individuals, depending on their particular circumstances. What might be a minor inconvenience for one person may have far reaching effects for another. Your reasons for not accepting treatment may not seem as important to your doctor as they do to you. Julie, who was diagnosed with breast cancer, was concerned that the possible side effects of radiotherapy treatment would affect the movement in her arm. Julie was a professional violinist, and restricted shoulder movement could limit her ability to continue playing. As well as losing an income, music was extremely important to Julie's quality of life. She decided against having radiotherapy treatment at that time. Naturally, doctors want to offer their patients the best chance of fighting their disease. However, there are no certain guarantees and, in the end, it is your body and your life.

Your decision to refuse treatment must be based on sufficient information that you understand and that you are aware of the consequences that might result from your decision. You also need to understand what alternative treatment options might be available. Whether or not you decide to accept treatment, it is important that you feel comfortable with the decision and have not been put under any sort of pressure by health professionals, family or friends. If, having weighed up all the pros and cons of a treatment, you decide you don't want to go ahead with it, talk through your concerns with your doctor. What happens next depends on the decision you make. For example, if you decide not to have any curative treatment, perhaps because you feel the risks outweigh the benefits, it doesn't mean that the doctors will wash their hands of you. There is always something that can be done. For example, there may be an alternative treatment with more acceptable risks or side-effects, although the benefits may not be as certain. Or you may be offered more frequent check-ups to monitor your progress. On the other hand, the focus of care may be on controlling any symptoms such as pain.

Sometimes people decline treatment because they do not fully understand the context in which it is being offered. John was offered steroids as part of an anti-sickness regime when he underwent chemotherapy treatment. His mother had had rheumatoid arthritis for which she had taken steroids over many years. John had seen some of the side effects of taking steroids long term and assuming they would also affect him, declined taking them. Health professionals should always question why an individual wants to decline a treatment, to allow the opportunity for a fuller discussion. Equally, it applies that you shouldn't make assumptions about how treatment may affect you, whether your experience is based on unrelated or similar circumstances.

While your doctor's priority is to offer you the most appropriate treatment available to help you get well, your own beliefs on treatment and your quality of life are just as important. Doctors will have to accept your decision *not* to receive treatment, provided they feel you are competent to make an informed decision.

How can I get the information I need to make a decision?

Having talked about the importance of having enough information to make your treatment decisions, how can you be sure that you have the right information in a form that you understand?

Most people say they find it difficult to take in and remember information when they are first told something shocking. So, when you are told you have cancer, even if this is what you have been expecting to hear, it will take you time to absorb everything that has been said. You may find it helpful to spend some time organising your thoughts, perhaps putting them down on paper. Your understanding at this time is likely to be a combination of your previous experience of illness and what you have read, heard or seen about cancer. There is no real substitute for exchanging information face-to-face during a consultation, where all individuals are contributing. When we have conversations with friends, for example, as well as listening to what they have to say we are also watching them. We are picking up non-verbal clues such as the way they are sitting, whether there is eye contact or what they are doing with their hands. This may not always be on a conscious level but body language combined with the words we hear both contribute to our interpretation of the words and our understanding of them. Studies have shown that some people only remember one tenth of what they were told during a consultation. Many people find that additional information they can return to in their own time is an essential back up to what they have been told. It can relieve some of the pressure of having to remember everything.

There is often a temptation to want as much information as possible as soon as possible. Using information as a way of coping is a strategy that many people find helpful. On the other hand, too much information at the beginning can be confusing until it starts to mean something. Often it is more helpful to have information in stages. If it is given at a point where it is likely to be understood, it is also more likely to be retained.

Sources of information

There is a wealth of cancer related information available. In addition to information from health professionals (both verbal and written), other sources include telephone helplines, written information from cancer charities; books, magazines and newspapers; television and radio; the Internet, family, friends and other people with cancer.

Seeking information from other sources helps many people feel they have pursued all their options before making a decision.

Health professionals should not see this as a negative reflection on what they are offering; they should recognise an individual's desire to retain some control in a situation that may otherwise seem to be spiralling out of control.

More information on information resources is covered in Chapter 10.

Conclusion

Having to cope with what may be months of treatment can be a daunting experience. Many people say that they feel they are on a roller coaster with the world spinning past them. There is so much to absorb that it is not surprising that many people feel they are losing control of their lives. But it doesn't have to be like this. There are many steps you can take to start regaining control of what is happening to you and to feel part of any decisions that are made. Of course, what is comfortable for one person may not necessarily feel right for another. Information can be a very valuable coping tool, but only if it is information you want, at a time when you want it. On its own, information may have limited use unless it is presented in a form that is easy to understand and digest. This is where you can influence what will be most helpful to you.

Remember:

- You can be in control of the amount of information you are given
- Always ask for another explanation if you don't understand something you are told
- Ask as many questions as you need in order to understand what you are being told

You will usually be given some time before you have to make any decisions.

Resources

The following addresses and websites are all good sources of information:

CancerBACUP
3 Bath Place, Rivington Street, London EC2A 3JR
Helpline 0808 800 1234
www.cancerbacup.org.uk
Cancer nurses provide information and emotional support on all aspects of cancer. They produce a wide range of booklets and fact sheets on cancer, its treatments and the practical issues of coping.

Cancer Research UK
PO Box 123, Lincoln's Inn Fields, London WC2A 3PX
Tel: 020 7242 0200
www.cancerhelp.org.uk
This website gives information about various aspects of cancer.

Commission for Health Improvement (CHI)
First Floor, Finsbury Tower, 103–105 Bunhill Row, London EC1Y 8TG
Tel: 020 7448 9200
www.chi.nhs.uk
CHI was established to improve the quality of patient care in the NHS by focusing on the experience of those using the services.

Consumers in NHS Research
Support Unit, Wessex House, Upper Market Street,
Eastleigh, Hampshire SO50 9FD
Tel: 023 8065 1088
www.conres.co.uk/lin.htm
Promoting consumer involvement in NHS research and development.

Department of Health (DoH)
www.doh.gov.uk/cancer
Government documents about cancer services.
www.doh.gov.uk/consent
Government documents about the consent process.

Department of Health Publications
PO Box 777, London SE1 6XH
Fax: 01623 724524
E-mail doh@prolog.uk.com
Tel: NHS Response Line on 08701 555 455
Please quote the title and reference number for each title wherever possible.

Macmillan Cancer Relief
89 Albert Embankment, London SE1 7UQ
Macmillan Cancerline: 0808 808 2020 (freephone)
www.macmillan.org.uk
Provides free information and support for people living with cancer.

National Institute for Clinical Excellence (NICE)
Midcity Place, High Holborn, London WC1V 6NA
Tel: 020 7067 5800
www.nice.org.uk
NICE provides guidance for healthcare professionals, and patients and their carers, that will help to inform their decisions about treatment and healthcare.

Royal Marsden
The Patient Information Service
Fulham Road, London SW3 6JJ
Tel: 020 7808 2831/2811
www.royalmarsden.org
The Royal Marsden's Patient Information Service produces a wide range of booklets on cancer, its treatments and the practical issues of coping.

6
Coping with cancer

Living successfully with the knowledge that you have cancer will put a whole new perspective on your life. A diagnosis of cancer is no longer an automatic death sentence, so increasing numbers of people are learning to live with cancer as a chronic illness. Some of these people use strategies that have proved successful in dealing with other life events to manage their cancer experience. However, these normal coping strategies are often tested. Cancer is likely to change how you relate to family and friends and it may challenge your relationships. Every person's experience of cancer will be unique to them.

> *It's a bit like a maze. Different people take different journeys through that maze. Therefore you can have people with exactly the same diagnosis but it depends on where they start off, how that first journey starts. The people they deal with, how the news is broken, how they deal with the support they have, you can't predict that. So in a way, everybody is on this big isolated journey and thinks they're the only person who's ever been on that journey.*
>
> **Caroline, breast cancer**

The word 'coping' refers to what we actually think and do in a particular situation, and how this helps us to manage that situation. It may be by overcoming, reducing or accepting the threat of the encounter. We assess what is at stake and then consider what coping resources and options are available to help us. Sometimes we may choose more active coping strategies such as seeking information, trying to get help, preventing things from happening, and taking direct action. Or we may use passive strategies to help us cope emotionally. These may include *avoiding* talking or thinking about the issue, cultivating a sense of *detachment* from it and blaming either others or ourselves. We all develop different ways of coping, depending on how we interpret a stressful situation and what we think will help us to avoid being harmed by it.

It is normal to strive for balance in our lives, but sometimes events overcome us and we find ourselves in crisis. The word 'crisis' implies a disaster or predicament, although we usually use the word to describe an unexpected or sudden turn of events that represents a threat. Bereavement, divorce, losing a job and illness are all examples of life crises.

There are typically four stages in the course of a crisis: the shock phase; the reaction phase; the working phase and the reorientation phase. Initially, many people may feel stunned when they are diagnosed with cancer. As shock sets in, the world can seem unreal. These reactions are protective mechanisms that people often use to help cope with the initial shock. They help to prevent us from being overwhelmed by such a situation. Following on from these kinds of reactions, people may start to think more constructively and start looking to the future. However, the way people deal with crisis situations is very individual. Not everyone will experience the stages described here, and some may find they move backwards and forwards between them. But if you are able to recognise your feelings and emotions, it can be easier to understand how to cope with them.

Just as there are many possible reactions to a diagnosis, there are many different coping strategies that can be used to help in a crisis situation. You may well find that you use different strategies at different times during your cancer experience.

The impact of cancer on you

Most people find that the experience of living with cancer alters their lives. Priorities often change when we realise that we aren't invincible. It can be a very positive opportunity to take stock of your life and to reflect on what is most important to you. Maybe this is the first time that you have been able to think about yourself for once and what you want out of life. It is all too easy to say, 'Well, I'd do that if only I had more time or when I retire'. It is such a shame when it takes something like cancer to trigger a reappraisal of who we are and what we are.

Not everyone, of course, will undergo major transformations. Change can be far subtler and may not even happen on a conscious level. Neither will change necessarily be instantaneous; it often takes place over a long period of time.

I was busy, busy, busy which was probably a way of coping. Not only busy at work because my social life was the same. I still have a very busy social life and enjoy periods on my own but I probably never sat and listened to

music and certainly didn't meditate or do any contemplative activities,
which I make sure I fit in now.

Anne, breast cancer

People increasingly find it difficult to make time for their own needs when they lead such busy lives. Perhaps you would think it was selfish to put yourself first. Looking after your own needs can be an important step in your recovery. This won't happen overnight but there are many ways in which you can start to think about how you want to live your life.

Although I've always been quite assertive and was never a doormat, I
would always say yes and now I don't.

Anne, breast cancer

The impact of cancer on the family

Cancer doesn't just affect the individual; it affects everyone around them. Our relationships with other people are important, particularly in a crisis. Just as you have to come to terms with an uncertain future, so do your family. They have to adjust to new, difficult emotions, as well as to changes in roles and routines. This may be the first time that family relationships have been put to the test. It is not surprising that communication sometimes breaks down. Family members may become very protective towards you, perhaps to avoid upsetting you. They may take on tasks around the home without thinking to ask if this is what you want. Often it is a way of coping with their own feelings. You are the one who has the illness and has to cope with the physical effects of treatment. It is not easy standing on the sidelines watching someone you care for go through this. Many people find it difficult to remain passive and react by taking control in some way. They may do this through seeking information, perhaps about different treatments, by wanting to be involved in decision making, or by taking over roles that have traditionally been yours.

Let your family know how you feel, both emotionally and physically. The more they know how you feel, the better they will be able to give you the support you want. You may not find this easy if your family has never been one to express emotions openly. Your family may also find it difficult to tell you how they feel. It is not uncommon for people to react angrily, because their lives as well as yours are changing and they may feel they have no control over this change. You need to remember that this is a reflection on the situation rather than on you. Any major life event can be threatening and unsettling, and cause feelings of losing control. The more honest you and your family are, the better the chance of you all working through this situation. Sharing fears and concerns will not necessarily make them go away, but it will help you feel you don't have to deal with them in isolation.

People react differently to stressful situations, depending on their personality and previous experiences. Their way of coping will also vary. Some people respond to difficult situations by taking refuge in their work. Others may focus their energies on family life or on social activities. Quite often this might come across as not caring or understanding the situation. All relationships have their ups and downs, and times when we are happy, sad or cross. It is all part of normal family life. It can feel uncomfortable complaining about work or a headache when these things seem so trivial compared to a life threatening illness. Family members may feel guilty that it is you who has the illness not them. However difficult it may be, talking about how you each feel will help you to understand each other and work through your different coping strategies.

My daughter was diagnosed with acute myeloid leukaemia when she was 36. She had always lived very independently and had to come back from abroad – where she was very happy – to be treated. I was her main 'carer' by choice, because her boyfriend was also abroad and she was being treated in a hospital near to where I lived.

It was a huge challenge to both of us to work out what she needed from me. And of course it varied from phase to phase of the illness, as well as with her current state of mind. The challenge for me as a person was to stay responsive, pick up on what was going on for her, and look after myself at the same time. I had to endlessly remind myself that although she was 'my little girl', she was centrally an adult who wanted to manage her illness in her own way, most of the time. As well as that, I needed to be ready for the times when she wanted to be supported, advised, and coddled. It was about the most maturing experience I've ever had.

You can imagine what it did to me, being alongside while she was in pain, scared, and very ill. I had to set all that aside in order to be reasonably strong for her. I didn't want her to worry about me when she had a lot to worry about herself. The communication between us was essential; and we got better and better at being truthful and tough where necessary.

There was a big question about when and whether her father or I should talk to her doctors. To begin with she was fierce about it being entirely her business. Later, when she wasn't so well, she wanted me to talk with them.

It seemed important to me that we shouldn't know more than she had been told; it was right that she had the power over what we knew about the illness from the doctors.

Keeping that clear seemed essential, and this included talking with friends and relations. She was very clear that she hated the thought of 'people talking about her' rather than talking direct to her.

One useful role I took was in talking to people who wanted to visit her but who she didn't particularly want to see. Her feeling was that if she wouldn't normally see them when she was in England, it didn't make sense to see them just because she was ill. I agreed with that and was happy to take the unpopular role of filtering the visitors according to what she wanted.

Judy (mother)

Be honest about what you want from your family. It is not always possible to predict how you will feel when you are having treatment. You may find that your life can continue much as it did before, or you may find it takes more out of you than you expected. Many people feel more tired than usual at some stage of their illness. This is perfectly normal and can take some adjusting to, especially for people who have always been active. If you get tired easily, focus your energies on the things you enjoy doing and ask for help with other tasks. Usually people are only too glad to help out in a positive way.

Coping during treatment

Often it is the little things that can create the most stress. Parking is a good example and is becoming a growing problem for hospitals.

As soon as you and your family are aware of your cancer diagnosis and it becomes likely that you will be incapacitated, apply for a disability badge. Contact your local council straightaway and fill out the relevant forms relating to disability. Macmillan nurses can help with filling out the relevant form and getting it signed by an oncologist or GP.

Regular visits to the hospital for me and my family became very costly and difficult in terms of finding a parking space. It takes time for the local authority to process your application for a disability badge. In my case, by the time it was actually issued I was two-thirds of the way through my chemotherapy. The sooner you apply the better.

Parking is one worry your family or yourself should not have to deal with at such an anxious time.

Nina, sarcoma

Genetics

Some people may find themselves having to confront questions about whether or not their cancer has a genetic origin. This may be because of their age when they developed cancer, the type of cancer or the fact that other members of the family have had cancer.

One of the most common questions a patient with cancer is asked is whether they have a family history. My registrar asked me very shortly after my diagnosis for a sarcoma. This question over family history or genes is one that people with cancer have to deal with over and over again, regardless of whether they choose to go for genetic testing or not. At the same time, it's astounding how even good friends will try and reassure themselves that the cause of your cancer was due to your family's weird genes. In fact it's surprising how very comfortable people are in telling you 'It's genetic' – an area which should require far greater sensitivity.

In my case, I only became interested in finding out if this really was true once I was in remission. Having your family branded 'a cancer family' is very painful and apart from the legal implications with regard to life insurance etc. it's not an easy thing to cope with.

My own need for genetic knowledge was increased when my mother was diagnosed with breast cancer soon after my own recovery. I was referred to a genetic oncologist who felt there might be a possible link between the breast cancer and the sarcoma.

When I returned to see the genetic oncologist three years later, my sister aged 40 had been diagnosed with breast cancer. This time I was supported from the start by a genetic counsellor and nurse and had my every concern taken seriously by the genetic oncologist. It was not just about helping out with their research as I had felt the first time. This time it was made more clear to me that the process of genetic testing is a very lengthy one – results are not given in a couple of weeks and can take over 6 – 8 months in the UK. It is a period of great anxiety if you feel a time bomb may be going off anytime. It was crucial that I was supported throughout and the process that was now in place was reassuring.

Fortunately, the results from the first time proved negative. I would have otherwise been very concerned about having more lethal cancers. A new blood sample was taken to determine whether I had genes that are linked to breast cancer. I also provided histology reports of members of my family back to the genetic department. A few months later, the genetic oncologist returned to me with the genetic probabilities of having these genes. I was then set up on hereditary breast cancer genetic screening programmes. I was also referred for additional counselling during this very anxious time.

Overall, the genetics team took great consideration and interest in my well being. Their support was more than encouraging. I was even sent documentation on using Tamoxifen as a prophylactic [i.e. to prevent breast cancer developing] *in the US and the comparisons with its use in the UK. Tamoxifen was another area of great anxiety for me. I did not want to take a drug, which would affect my fertility, cause the early onset of the menopause and other side effects. The closer screening suggested, instead put my mind at rest.*

Genetic knowledge in my case was vital and it allowed me to deal with my fears. The additional counselling and support given as part of the testing process allowed me to come to terms with some of the wider implications. Overall, knowing if I carry the breast cancer genes helps me with decisions, for example, relating to hormone therapies, contraceptives and even IVF treatment. Oestrogens can especially increase the risk of breast cancer and ovarian cancer in a person with a genetic disposition. Having this knowledge helped me decide how best to manage my lifestyle and diet.

Nina, sarcoma

Cancer genetic counselling is available for any individual who is concerned about their cancer risk. Families where there have been cases of cancer in young people, and families where several members have developed cancer may need genetic advice. If you are concerned, you should discuss this with either your oncologist or your GP, and ask to be referred through your nearest Regional Genetics Centre.

The impact of cancer on friends

The period after your diagnosis can be a testing time for friendships. Many people find friends don't always respond in the way they had expected. Even close friends may find it difficult to know what to say and what they should do. Again, their response will be influenced by their previous experience of cancer, and the fears and feelings it brings about. They may have minimal knowledge about cancer and not realise that it doesn't automatically mean a death sentence or that you can't catch it. If your friendship has been based on shared interests and activities, perhaps they worry that you will no longer be able to share them. When people don't know what to say, it can often be easier to avoid being in a situation where they risk saying the wrong thing. Withdrawing in this way can be very hurtful. Friends may be waiting for you to take the initiative about meeting up. Alternatively, friends may go to the other extreme and constantly ask you how you are and want to know all the details to the exclusion of any other conversation. Tell people if you prefer not to talk about your illness at a particular time, you don't always have to feel up to talking. This can be very tiring and you may need to gently remind them that you are still the same person you were before your diagnosis. Just because you are also living with cancer, doesn't mean that you can't continue to laugh together or argue about world events. Most importantly, it doesn't mean that you have ceased to be you!

While illness may strengthen some relationships, others fall by the wayside. Telling friends can be physically wearing when you are telling the same story over and over again.

I've actually lost a lot of friends through having cancer. I have become estranged from a very old friend because we no longer have anything in common. We speak on the 'phone, just socially, but she's not interested in the things that are going on in my life, and I can't relate to the things going on in hers. I mourn the loss of that friendship, very, very much. There have been a couple of casualties like that and I really mourn those but then new people have come into my life to give me great joy. So it's been a time of huge change and it's still going on.

Anne, breast cancer

Often people find that new friends enter their lives, or acquaintances develop into close friends. Most friends will want to help you in any way they can but may be unsure as to how they can best help. People who have been in this situation say that it can be helpful to make a list of things friends can do to help. This may include, for example, offers of lifts to the hospital or help with shopping and childcare. It can be easy to underestimate just how much help you may need, especially if you live on your own. Often it is little things that become difficult to cope with.

When it comes to practical help, it takes energy to have to think about what you want doing. A neighbour suggested coming in and changing my bed linen once a week and emptying my rubbish. Those were two very practical things that I couldn't do. Another friend picked up a load of shopping every week for about six weeks. It was wonderful. And somebody else came in and put the washing machine on and somebody else came and walked my dog. So you need the right form of support and then you get yourself organised. When you've just had a mastectomy, you can't even lift a kettle. You can't fill a kettle and hold it, so you're even doing things like filling a kettle with a cup. I can imagine anybody who's had abdominal surgery not being able to lift things. So it's the thoughtful things like making a bed and emptying the rubbish, they don't think of, when somebody says what can they do.

Anne, breast cancer

The impact of cancer on employment

Many people continue to work during their treatment, depending on the type of employment they have. At some stage, you are likely to be faced with explaining to your employer why you need to take time off or attend hospital appointments. Although you are not obliged to disclose your diagnosis, you may want to think through how you would deal with explaining any obvious physical changes. These may be a result of the illness itself or its treatment. You may find it helpful to talk with your doctor about how your treatments might affect your ability to do your job. Radiotherapy is likely to involve daily visits to the treatment centre. You may not experience any side effects at the start, but later on in your treatment you may start to feel more tired than usual. You may find that you can continue to work around your hospital appointments. If you have a physical job, your employer may be able to offer you alternative work that is less physically demanding while you are undergoing treatment. With chemotherapy, you may find that your treatment is every three weeks, for example, and that you feel unwell for only a couple of days. Therefore, you may find it helpful to take a day or two off when you have your treatment. There are no hard and fast rules, and what works for one person may not necessarily work for another. Taking time off at the time when you need it, rather than struggling on, can be beneficial in the long run.

There are also other strategies that you might wish to consider if you continue working:

- Coming into work later and going home earlier to avoid the rush hour traffic
- Working at home (if appropriate)
- Working part time
- Changing to alternative work until you have fully recovered.

Whether or not you tell your work colleagues your diagnosis is a decision only you can make. It is human nature to speculate when there are changes to a normal routine and you may decide that you prefer your colleagues to know something about what is going on. Some people have said that they found it easier for their manager to give basic information to their colleagues. This doesn't mean to say that your colleagues need to know all the intimate details, but it might be helpful for you if they know enough to understand why you might be absent or tire more easily. During treatment that might cause hair loss (and it is important to remember that not all treatment does), you may be faced with the decision of whether or not to wear a wig. Some people find wearing a wig helps keep some semblance of normality while others prefer not to wear one – this is very much down to personal preference. Just as family and friends can find it difficult to know what to say, so may your colleagues. Don't feel you have to talk about any aspect of your illness if you don't want to.

You may have a colleague who has been through a similar experience – and it can be helpful if you are working with someone who understands something of what you are going through. Some people find that colleagues they didn't know very well before turn out to have had cancer and are now living full lives again.

However, all experiences are individual and your journey will be different from anyone else's journey.

My world was turned upside down by my cancer diagnosis. The more I thought about it the more I felt I must reappraise my life and what I was doing. Not so much my marriage, though I could have imagined that being part of my thinking about what needed changing if it was not so loving and supportive, but much more my work. At the time I was a social worker, in a very stressful sector of the profession – child protection; and I had a caseload of the complex cases, as I was a senior social worker. Often, I was in the High Court giving evidence or investigating abuse of children. After 10 years I was beginning to find it stressful. I had ideas of leaving, but I was stuck and I had no idea what a career move would hold. I had trained as a family therapist some years before and knew it would take time to build up a client base.

Suddenly, my mind was made up. I would leave social work and begin as a family therapist. I needed to do it otherwise my wish to find fulfilment would pass me by. We had no mortgage by then and thank goodness our financial position was relatively secure. Had this not been so I would have become seriously depressed I am sure.

Cancer does force change upon people. Sometimes it is not so negative. I found I stepped out of the rat-race of highly pressurised local government services beleaguered by staff cuts, greater expectations on those left, more and more regulation, restructuring and reorganisations that bewildered everyone because they completely lacked consideration for the employees who had to make it all work and I stepped into a world that I could control much more, where I was in charge of my timetable and weekly structure. My immediate family saw me more.

Mark, sarcoma

What if the cancer returns?

Good communication is vital whenever difficult news is given, not just at diagnosis. At every stage, the necessary information needs to be conveyed in a sensitive way, especially when decisions need to be made.

Two of my most memorable communication experiences have been with doctors working, not in oncology, but in a hospital blood pressure clinic. Having asked me many details about my cancer history, the first of these doctors looked me straight in the eye and said, 'The problems you've been left with are a small price to pay for having survived'. I'm not often lost for words, but I was half way home on the bus before an appropriate response came to mind!

The second doctor could not have been more different. Some routine testing had discovered that I had metastatic spread of my cancer ['secondaries'], which was a bolt from the blue, since I'd not had any symptoms of this. I was recalled to the clinic, where this unfortunate doctor had the task of breaking the bad news to me – not an everyday situation in the blood pressure clinic.

He put down his pen, pushed the paperwork to the back of the desk, turned his chair to face me and gave me his undivided attention. Not only that, but he found the right words to say and, in every way, showed me the utmost respect. He ended by saying, 'I have tremendous admiration for the way in which you are dealing with this'. Sometimes people say that sort of thing and it just sounds patronising, but not on this occasion.

Karen, breast cancer

However difficult it is to hear that initial diagnosis of cancer, learning of a recurrence can be worse than the first time round. When the initial shock wears off after cancer is first diagnosed, there may be many constructive thoughts and actions to bring about hope. Treatment plans are discussed and decisions made – all positive actions, taking you towards a future. Family – and friends too – can rally round with support. A recurrence of your initial cancer, or the spread of cancer to other parts of the body ('metastases' or 'secondaries') will test the coping and communication skills of everyone concerned. At such times support is crucial.

> *Having cancer is very isolating and discovering I had secondary cancer added to the feeling of isolation. It takes a great deal of strength to make rational and considered choices when one is in pain both physically and mentally, and it is at times like this that one realises how vital communication is. Strength does come from within but it is helped considerably by talking to and having support from people around you. Being able to talk about having cancer lessens the pressure and makes the illness more manageable. Managing cancer is an ongoing process but I know, through verbal and non-verbal communication I have as much support as I need from family, friends and cancer care professionals.*
>
> **Pamela, breast cancer**

This is often the time when many people re-evaluate their lives. When Anne finished treatment after her first diagnosis, she went back to work and put it out of her mind. It wasn't until she had a recurrence of her cancer, that she reflected that it had never occurred to her that she needed to look at her lifestyle. People may feel that whatever coping strategies they used at first, they were not actually enough.

> *I wouldn't say cancer was a turning point in that sense for me because I loved my life. It was pretty good and if I hadn't become ill, I'd have probably carried on that way. I was going to take early retirement anyway, so I think I'd have changed my life then. But I had to retire earlier for all sorts of reasons.*
>
> *I chose the things that I believed would improve my chances of staying alive. So I changed my diet. I've not become a vegan or a vegetarian but I've changed my diet in a lot of important ways that made me feel that I'm putting less toxins into my system through what I eat. So I'm giving my immune system a chance to deal with any secondaries that are developing. Having enough sleep and not being tired all the time; I was tired all the time.*
>
> **Anne, breast cancer**

Resources

CancerBACUP
3 Bath Place, Rivington Street, London EC2A 3JR
Tel: 020 7696 9003
Cancer Information Service: 0808 800 1234 (freephone)
www.cancerbacup.org.uk
Cancer nurses provide information and emotional support on all aspects of cancer. They produce a wide range of booklets and fact sheets on cancer, its treatments and the practical issues of coping.

Useful reading

Challenging Cancer (2002) Maurice Slevin & Nira Kfir, Class Publishing, London. ISBN: 1 85959 068 3

7
What you can do to help yourself? Support and complementary therapies

The last chapter looked at the different ways people cope with a diagnosis of cancer and how it can affect the people around you. At some stage, you may wonder what you can do to help yourself. There are many approaches you can follow to help you manage your experience of cancer in a caring and supportive way. This chapter explores the types of support that are available and the different types of complementary therapies.

Support

Cancer can be a lonely experience whether you are part of a loving family or live on your own. As much as family and friends often provide the main support network for many people, there are times when additional support can be invaluable. People often underestimate how much support they need and however close you may be to your family or friends, they may not always appear to understand the fears and anxieties you are dealing with. It is not easy for family and friends to know what to say or how they can best support you. You are not expected to cope with cancer on your own. People often find they experience a wide range of emotions, and, however supportive family and friends are, there may be times when you feel it would be helpful to talk to someone else. This could be a counsellor or you may, perhaps, prefer to talk to someone who has been through a similar experience who can understand what you're going through.

Counselling has helped me appreciate that there are many facets to my being that are strong, able, inspiring and creative. I have realised I have a passion for life that I did not fully appreciate before and the power of fear and uncertainty that cancer brought is not so overwhelming. Sometimes I do feel fragile and bewildered but at the same time I have never been more vital. My senses seem to be intensified; I absorb the rich details of the environment around me with piquancy and clarity. I am enjoying the moment but also planning for the future and I have a positive drive for life.

Pamela, breast cancer

The turning point for many people is when they acknowledge to themselves that they are living with cancer. Phrases such as 'joining the club' and identifying oneself as 'living with cancer' indicate the necessity to adapt to the concept of having cancer.

It wasn't really until I came out of hospital, even though I knew I had cancer, that I wanted to identify myself as being part of a community of people living with cancer and look at alternative support. If you think about different communities in life, there's a community living with HIV, a community of single mothers and there are lots of other things you're prepared to identify as. I was prepared to identify myself as a single mother, as a health professional, as a woman. But I wasn't, in the early stages, prepared to identify myself as someone living with cancer and I didn't want to go to a support group or centre.

Sadie, colon cancer

These turning points suggest that once an individual reaches this stage, they are in a better position to make the most of the information and support available to them.

To begin with, I was still getting over this 'joining the club' bit and I didn't want to be in with a group of people with cancer. When I eventually went to the Bristol Cancer Help Centre, it was a real turning point, a wonderful experience. I was able to discover complementary therapies that helped me.

Anne, breast cancer

Hospital-based support

Many oncology departments recognise the need for support and provide counsellors and psychologists to help people deal with emotional and psychological issues. Support groups run by hospital staff are also becoming more common in many areas. Some of these are for people affected by any type of cancer, while others are set up for particular groups, such as people with lung cancer. These groups can provide excellent access to hospital staff in a more informal setting than the clinic or treatment unit, thus offering relaxed opportunities for questions to be asked and concerns clarified.

Community-based support

Meeting and talking with others in a similar position can be invaluable for some people. Community-based support and self-help groups can take a number of forms. Many local support groups are run by volunteers with personal experience as patients or carers, sometimes with voluntary input from health professionals. These groups may hold an open meeting monthly or more often, sometimes with a speaker. Some may also have other activities such as a telephone helpline, help with transport, or hospital visits.

People join support groups for many reasons, including:
- To find others with similar experiences;
- To be able to talk about what has happened and is still happening, to people with a sympathetic ear who are in a position to understand;
- To find practical information and advice – for instance about insurance issues, how people cope with treatments, ways people have found of coping, which local organisations offer help and of what kind (such as transport or help with shopping);
- In order to regain a sense of choice and control, of being able to have a say in determining what is happening in their life;
- To stop feeling isolated and afraid, and to develop a sense of solidarity with others;
- To feel like an individual again.

Paradoxically, by having a place where it is acceptable to talk a lot about the cancer experience, people are often freed to move beyond it, and to pursue other interests in life.

Cancer support and resource centres

In some places there are community-based centres that are open throughout the week, offering a wide range of services. These may include support groups; classes and workshops on topics such as yoga, relaxation or nutrition; one-to-one complementary therapies and counselling; and information on many practical aspects of cancer, such as benefits advice and travel insurance. The services are available to carers, family members and friends of people with cancer. These centres have permanent staff, and are run in a professional manner, normally offering supervision and support to practitioners and staff.

> *Having finished treatment, I had the feeling of being all alone until I started to go back to the Cancer Resource Centre. Meeting other people in the 'self discovery group' and listening to their stories, I thanked my lucky stars that I was not that badly off after all. Making things at the 'creative art therapy' class was something I looked forward to with great anticipation. The centre is starting a new class for writers, artists and musicians and I hope to take up painting and drawing. Attending the centre has certainly helped me to improve the quality of my life and my thinking about learning to live with cancer.*
>
> **David, breast cancer**

Complementary therapies

There is growing interest in the use of complementary therapies to help people cope with cancer. You may want to find out more about the different complementary therapies available, which ones will be most helpful and how to find a suitable practitioner.

Complementary therapies offer a holistic approach to care and treat the whole person, not just the illness. They should not be seen as an alternative to conventional medical treatment, but rather as something that can be used in addition. This is in contrast to alternative therapies that may make claims to cure cancer.

Many people find that using one or more of the complementary therapies can be extremely helpful, especially while they are coping with the effects of treatment. It is all too easy to feel that you have little control over what happens to you and using complementary therapies can help you to feel that you are doing something positive to help yourself.

Doctors are becoming increasingly aware that the psychological and emotional support people gain from complementary therapy helps them to live with cancer. Some oncology departments are able to offer a limited range of therapies such as counselling or massage so it's worth asking what is available in your hospital. It is also worth asking your GP, as some practices may have complementary therapists working there. Another place where complementary therapies are often available is your local cancer support centre. If you used a particular therapy before you were diagnosed, you may find that you can continue to use it as well as exploring other therapies. Often people only come to complementary therapies for the first time during their cancer experience and are directed to them by nurses and other patients.

A colleague had been helped enormously by going to the Bristol Cancer Help Centre and so I eventually booked. It was a real turning point; a wonderful experience. I was able to discover complementary therapies that helped me. I had spiritual healing; I talked to a counsellor and discovered useful things to explore. The counsellor persuaded me to go along to her support group in London.

Anne, breast cancer

Choosing a private therapist should be approached carefully. You should ensure that they are registered with a recognised professional organisation, if appropriate, and that they have experience of working with people undergoing cancer treatment. Many therapies can work out expensive if used on a regular basis. So it is important that you choose a therapy that feels right for you and that you don't feel under any pressure from friends and family to try something that makes you feel uncomfortable.

The Institute for Complementary Medicine and The Prince of Wales Foundation for Integrated Health provide information for the public on complementary medicine and details of practitioners (see *Resources*). You could also ask friends for recommendations.

A useful website, developed by doctors and specialists is www.whole healthmd.com. Although it is an American site, it guides you through different complementary therapies, covering what each therapy is; how it works; what you can expect; health benefits; how to choose a practitioner (although this relates to American practice, it does give useful guidance) and cautions.

As there are a large number of different complementary therapies, it may be helpful to describe some of the more common therapies you are most likely to come across. Some of these therapies may help you to cope better with symptoms and others may encourage a sense of well-being. Let your doctor know that you are receiving some form of complementary therapy, and your therapist know that you have cancer. Occasionally there may be a therapy that is not suitable for a particular type of cancer or during a particular treatment.

Physical therapies

Physical therapies use touch and in addition to holistic massage, there are other therapies involving massage techniques such as aromatherapy, reflexology and shiatsu. Massage has been used for a long time and involves working on the muscles to release excess tension, which helps relaxation. It also stimulates the circulation of blood and lymph around the body, to encourage the removal of waste products and toxins. While the benefits of a therapy such as massage are no longer disputed, a therapist should avoid massaging an area that is being treated with radiotherapy for example.

Aromatherapy is often used in conjunction with massage and involves the use of essential oils distilled from flowers, herbs, roots and leaves. The essential oils are blended in a carrier oil. You can also use the essential oils outside the session, for example, in baths and oil burners. During chemotherapy and radiotherapy treatment, the skin may be more sensitive than usual, so care needs to be taken with using essential oils. If you are receiving chemotherapy, you may find your sense of smell is affected and an essential oil that you would normally find agreeable becomes unpleasant.

Reflexology is an ancient form of Chinese medicine using touch but the therapist works only on the feet and/or hands. It is based on the belief that organs and tissues in the body are connected with reflex points on the feet or hands. Massage on these points affects the corresponding part of the body and a deep sense of relaxation is often felt throughout the body after a session.

Holistic therapies

The aim of holistic therapies is to treat the whole person, not just the symptoms. Acupuncture has its origins in Traditional Chinese Medicine (TCM), which is concerned with preventing and treating disease. Traditional Chinese Medicine believes that 'Chi' or energy flows through a network of meridians or channels in the body. When these energy channels become blocked, health problems can occur. Acupuncture involves inserting fine, sterile needles into specific points in the body to unblock these channels and free energy. It has been found to help relieve pain and some of the side effects of chemotherapy. Although the training for acupuncture does not require a medical background, some medical doctors undergo further training in acupuncture. Ask your GP or hospital doctor if you would like to be referred to a medical acupuncturist.

Herbal medicine involves the use of the whole plant (roots, leaves, stem and seed) to treat illnesses and maintain health. Medicines are given to improve the body's natural functions and to restore a natural balance of health. Herbal medicines can be given in many forms, such as liquids, infusions, tablets and local preparations. Herbalists may practice Western herbalism or be practitioners of Traditional Chinese Medicine, also offering acupuncture. It is a good idea to tell your doctor if you are considering herbal medicines in case they work against other medicines you are already taking.

Homoeopathy is a system of treatment developed from the belief that 'like is cured by like'. Homoeopaths prescribe remedies containing a diluted form of a substance that produces similar effects to those of the illness. There are five homoeopathic hospitals and some of them offer a complementary cancer care programme that you can use alongside your hospital treatment. It is not an alternative to conventional medical treatment. Ask your doctor if you can be referred to their clinic if you are interested. There are also professional homoeopaths who are not medical doctors.

Healing therapies

With healing, the healer is a channel through which healing energy can pass to the client and this sometimes involves touch. Healing can be re-energising and relaxing. It helps them make the most of their own healing abilities, to cope with illness, injury or stress. Many people say that they experience a deep sense of relaxation and peace after a healing session. You do not need to have 'faith', as healing is not associated with any particular religion. Reiki is another form of healing thought to originate from the healing practices of ancient Tibetan monks.

'Thinking' therapies

'Thinking' therapies or mind-body therapies can all be practised on their own or in a group, although you may find it helpful to find a teacher to take you through the techniques. These are therapies that you can do to make yourself feel better. There is an overlap between some of the following therapies – choose the one that you feel most comfortable with. They can all help with reducing stress

Meditation is a technique used to reach a state of mental and physical tranquillity. There are many forms of meditation, most of them originating in the East. You sit in a comfortable position either in a chair or on the floor, with your eyes closed. Meditation focuses on the mind and through concentration, you can control your thoughts. This has a relaxing effect on the body. Concentrating on your breathing can help you to focus your thought and ignore distractions. Meditation needs to be practised on a regular basis to gain long-term benefits.

Relaxation is an active process that you need to think about and it involves the mind as well as the body. Many people say they find it hard to relax and it is helpful to work with a therapist or use special audiotapes to lead you into a state of relaxation.

Guided imagery or visualisation is similar to meditation and relaxation in that you start with breathing or relaxation exercises first. You may find it helpful to be led through creative visualisation exercises, which uses images or pictures to create positive images in the mind. Once you have learnt the technique of visualisation, you can practice it at home. Relaxation and visualisation exercises are useful techniques to help counteract side effects of cancer treatments such as nausea and vomiting, or pain.

Creative art or art therapy encourages people to express their feelings without having to use words through working with art materials. This can involve different techniques such as drawing, painting or modelling. You don't have to be able to 'draw' as this therapy focuses on the creation of a piece of work rather than the end product. Art therapy may be offered individually or in groups. Some people find it helpful to talk through with the therapist what their work might be saying about their experiences or feelings.

I was in shock for about one year and I couldn't find anything that made me feel better. Writing helped to an extent but it was art therapy that helped me come to terms with cancer.

Alison, colon cancer

Creative writing involves putting thoughts and feelings onto paper. This may be in the form of keeping a diary or perhaps writing a letter to someone, that may never be sent. Again, you don't have to be a 'writer' but many people say they find it helpful to express feelings on paper they may find difficult to say face-to-face.

Diet and nutrition
Food plays an important role in lives and not surprisingly, many people are interested in the link between diet and cancer. There is plenty of evidence that a healthy balanced diet can have a protective role in preventing cancer. However, there is no conclusive evidence to date to support the claims

made by alternative diets, although some individuals report positive outcomes from following them. More research into different dietary approaches is needed. Certainly some people feel much better following a rigorous nutritional regime, but not everyone will feel a benefit.

Cancer and its treatments such as chemotherapy and radiotherapy can have an effect on appetite and the enjoyment of food for many people. Eating well during treatment is an important part of the healing process and this is not a good time to lose too much weight. If you are experiencing any difficulties with eating, for example, loss of appetite, feeling sick, a sore mouth, you may want to see a dietitian. Hospital dietitians, who are state registered, can provide advice about diet based on scientific evidence. You can also talk to them about nutritional supplements.

Nutritional therapists are not state registered and their training is not regulated, which can make it difficult to know if they are giving sound advice. Their emphasis with cancer is on boosting the immune system.

The Bristol Cancer Help Centre has a special interest in nutrition and cancer. Their programme focuses on developing a healthy approach to eating which can be maintained after treatment has finished. They advise a diet that avoids red meat and dairy produce, and is low in fat, caffeine, sugar and salt, preservatives and additives, smoked or pickled foods. Herb and fruit teas are advised rather than tea and coffee.

Macrobiotics takes a holistic approach to healing and health, and diet is part of this philosophy. Based on ancient Chinese beliefs, a macrobiotic diet aims to provide a balance between the yin foods, which are female, darker, cooler and moister and yang foods, which are male, lighter, warmer and drier. The diet is mainly vegan and includes organic 50 per cent wholegrain cereals and 20-30 per cent fresh vegetables. We all have yin and yang qualities and therefore macrobiotic diets need to be planned around individual needs.

Often it is after treatment has finished that people become interested in diet, to give their body the best chance for recovery. Specific diets do not appeal to everyone and you may prefer to follow a healthy eating plan and ensure that you have a good balance between the different types of foods. This may mean cutting down on red meat and fat, and aiming for five portions of fruit and vegetables a day.

It is a good idea to check the suitability of alternative, complementary diets or nutritional supplements that claim to influence the outcome of cancer with a dietitian or your doctor. As with all therapies, it is a matter of personal choice and must suit your lifestyle; any potential benefit must outweigh any potential burden.

Moving on when treatment has finished

Cancer is likely to have changed your life in many ways and finishing treatment becomes a time to look forward to the future. Now you can start recovering emotionally and physically. People often assume that life will return to normal rapidly, and are bewildered when recovery seems to be slow.

> *Once treatment is over often people feel the illness is now over. In fact, it can take a lot longer to come to terms with the experience and the tiredness of treatment. It is important to make this clear to friends even if you believe it is now all finally over. I only realised this in retrospect. Also, often people save up their own frustrations with your illness for when the treatment is completely over. It can all be very overwhelming after recovery.*
>
> **Nina, sarcoma**

Life during your treatment may have been very full, coping with various appointments, treatments and side effects. You may have focused all your energy on just getting through each day. It can also be a time for reflection, to make sense of the experience you have undergone. Individuals are ready for information at different stages and many people find they are often more able to receive and understand information after their treatment has finished.

> *. . . there are two sets of information that you need at different stages. Stuff to help you get through the treatment on a day to day basis and the more global information that helps you understand your symptoms in your body and helps you to make sense of that.*
>
> **Sadie, colon cancer**

This may be a time when you find that you can cope with a greater understanding of what has been happening to you in order to prepare for the future. The need for support does not disappear once treatment has finished, as it is often later on that the lack of support is felt so keenly. People talk about being bereft of support, abandoned or feeling vulnerable once their treatment had finished. Often a different kind of support structure is needed for the first year or two after finishing treatment.

It is also a time when you may think more about the possibility of recurrence. It is natural to worry that any little ache or pain is a sign that your cancer is returning. During treatment, you probably had regular contact with health professionals and the opportunity to talk through any anxieties. You may not find it so easy to know which health professional you can now talk to about your fears. Some people find their GP helpful and supportive while others are able to contact a health professional such as the nurse specialist in between follow-up appointments. If you are concerned about a symptom that doesn't go away, it is important that you tell someone. Uncertainty can be just as difficult to live with as being given bad news.

Long term effects of having had cancer

Increasingly, people are surviving cancer. This can raise a whole new set of needs for specific information and good communication. You may find you want to know about the long-term side effects of treatment. What about your future fertility? Women may be concerned about whether they will have an early menopause, and men may worry about lost sexual potency. Issues such as this can seem very remote early on, while you are having treatment for a life-threatening disease. But it is not enough to be told that survival is worth it at any cost. Quality of life is extremely important, and is closely entwined with both physical and psychological wellbeing. Few people will be untouched by their cancer experience, and many find ways of channelling their responses to it towards personal growth and development.

Living with cancer is very individual and no two people will share exactly the same experience. The following stories are the reflections on the cancer experiences of three individuals and convey the different realities that have emerged for each of them.

Patricia's story:

I was diagnosed with Hodgkin's disease in 1981, when I was 32. I had my spleen removed and six months of chemotherapy as an outpatient. I decided not to have radiotherapy. I also used a number of complementary approaches including visualisation, counselling and healing.

It is fortunate that there is a very good cure rate for Hodgkin's disease, and I haven't had any recurrences. Even though Hodgkin's disease is surrounded by far less uncertainty than most forms of cancer, the experience of having it changed my life forever.

Firstly, it made me aware that anything could happen at any time, with no clear cut reasons for it. I was in a very positive phase of my life at the time when the diagnosis occurred, and had done a great deal of therapy, self awareness work and received massage over a considerable period. I therefore didn't have the kind of experience that many describe, in which cancer is seen a turning point, giving permission to explore uncharted territories. While some people who get cancer at an early age say they know exactly what the predisposing factors were, I did not have that sense at all. The experience has left me with an acute sense of unpredictability.

Secondly, it taught me not to be one-sided in my view of things. Prior to this experience, I assumed that gentle, natural healing approaches were superior to orthodox medicine. Since orthodox medicine was essential to my recovery, I realised that it had a vital role in some situations, and that even though all cancer treatments tend to be tough to undergo, they could be the best option. This made me more inclined in the longer term not to assume that all the right is on any one side. I have often been in bridge-building roles in my career since that point, and the cancer experience prepared me for this.

Thirdly, since having chemotherapy, I have been inclined to put on weight, and not to be able to lose weight through cutting out things like sugar. This has led to me having a more difficult relationship with my body. In addition, I believe through some hormonal change as a result of the chemotherapy, I have had a big reduction in sexual energy, which has resulted in a loss of vitality within my personal (though not professional) life. This is one area where the communication from the medical team was less than honest. I was very concerned about the potential for losing fertility, and was told that that affected men not women. I wasn't told until I had completed the chemotherapy that it could bring on an early menopause. Because I hadn't been told this, I felt I hadn't been able to make that choice consciously, which then left me with a sense of loss. This was strange, since in other respects my consultant realised that I was the kind of person who was going to look into all the options, and he gave me time to consider whether to go ahead with the treatments proposed, and said that if I didn't opt clearly for these, there would be difficulty later if something went wrong.

Fourthly, I experienced the diagnosis and treatment of Hodgkin's disease as an 'initiation experience', in which a wound later becomes a source of creativity. I have founded and developed many services and initiatives for people with cancer and their carers in the twenty one years since my diagnosis, and this is a way of turning the strong emotional responses generated by a cancer experience into a creative force.

Fifthly, although in one sense having had an illness like cancer at an early age cuts you off from your contemporaries, in another way it creates connections with others who have had similar experiences, and increases empathy with people who experience other kinds of shocks and traumas.

Patricia's experience highlights the importance of having the right information at the right time. Halfway through or at the end of treatment, is not the time to learn of side effects such as fertility that will impact on the rest of your life. A sense of control over your destiny can be invaluable.

Mark's story:

I remember thinking, if this is so life-threatening, then I have to do something with my life. I was working for a local authority and found it stultifying. As a professional I had far too much administration to do. Our admin staff had been cut and cut and cut till we were sharing a typing pool with four other departments. Reports dictated or handwritten took over a month to return. I decided not to return after my surgery. I took the full amount of sick leave and applied for sickness retirement but was refused. So, I resigned. I had other skills to fall back on. I found work, sessional work and was my own boss. It was liberating though a bit frightening not to have to go to an office every day and report to managers and so on.

My surgery was successful. After months of waiting I heard that all the sarcoma was removed, and that it was low grade throughout. This meant it had not become uncontrolled, or that was my understanding, and had not spread. I had three-monthly checks that have now become six-monthly.

I enjoyed a long period of euphoria following the surgery. This might have been due to the after effects of the anaesthetic but I think it was mostly due to the decision I made to leave my job. Friends were astounded that I was so jolly and upbeat. I must have been rather poor company before if they noticed my change of mood as such a significant event. I have cancer to thank for that. Rather an extraordinary thing to claim, being pleased for having cancer. But I am convinced that without cancer I would have been cheerless and depressed, in a soul-destroying job, eroding my relationships with my wife and children, stuck in a rut and waiting for retirement.

I became involved in my local cancer services network, with the user-professional partnership. It keeps me in touch with how others cope with their cancers. The chair of our partnership died, quite unexpectedly. Well, unexpectedly for me. It was some impact and brought home to me that the deal one gets from cancer is unfairly distributed. I feel sometimes that my life and work is well balanced. It feels quite vibrant and healthy. My dad died recently. I was bereaved, understandably, but not defeated. He was 82; not so old. He'd had a tough life and was argumentative to the end. Thinking about him years ago and the likelihood of him dying made me wonder what it would feel like when it happened. Now I know what it's like. I would not have believed the change in my circumstances when it came about. I think I have coped with it well. Things came to a stop for a while but they're picking up now.

For Mark, the experience of cancer had a constructive outcome. It enabled him to turn to other skills he possessed in order to make a living. The sadness for many people, is that it takes an experience like cancer to liberate them from the less satisfying elements of their lives. Of course though, cancer is not going to be a positive experience for everyone. It can be a deeply distressing time, particularly if you feel you have everything to look forward to and a lifetime ahead in which to achieve your ambitions and dreams. Lucy's account is an honest reflection on her experience of having had cancer and the mixed emotions that can emerge as a result.

Lucy's story:

Some people say that having cancer turned out to be the best thing that happened to them. Well I couldn't disagree more, and it concerns me that such statements are creating new cancer myths, which can cause just as much damage as the old ones that cancer is contagious and always gets you in the end. Positive, life-enhancing things can and do come out of an experience of cancer and, people like me, go on to have children and resume happy, healthy, 'normal' lives. But it is not a walk in the park. Cancer is a deeply unpleasant and insidious disease and I don't think we are doing anyone any favours in trying to 'protect' them from this. Cancer – even when you recover from it – involves loss, pain, fear, tiredness, tedium and recovering from it took time and energy away from all the other things I wanted to be doing with my life. It concerns me that the pressure to be positive and upbeat about cancer can add to the stress of dealing with it.

Personally I found the worst time with cancer was after all the treatment had finished. The initial shock was huge, but I was being very positive, all my friends and family rallied round and the nature of shock itself helped so I couldn't take it all in at once. All during treatment there was support from health professionals as well as family and friends, also part of me was still numb and I was preoccupied with just getting through my treatments. It was afterwards when life started to get more back to 'normal' and hospital visits became routine follow-ups, friends and family thought I was OK now treatment was over, the prognosis was excellent . . . what did I have to worry about? It was then, over the following few months, that the accumulated tiredness, tension and terror of it all set in and I experienced severe anxiety, panic attacks and depression. Apparently it is relatively common to experience difficulties once treatment has ended, I wish someone had told me earlier, I couldn't understand what was happening to me. I felt guilty for being depressed when I had a good prognosis and a happy life, friends and family didn't understand what was happening either, we just all expected that I would bounce straight back in to normal life where I had left it. We couldn't have been more wrong.

My first thought on finding out I had cancer was 'Am I going to die soon'. My second concern, having been reassured about the first, was 'Will I still be able to have children'. My breast cancer was invasive, but caught at an early stage, so I had lumpectomy, radiotherapy and Tamoxifen. The Tamoxifen was most worrying in terms of my fertility as it caused premature menopause and ovarian cysts, and we didn't know at the time if this was permanent or not. Additionally, medical advice at that time was to stay on Tamoxifen for five years, but after two years I stopped taking it to try for a baby. Both my husband and I wanted children and felt strongly and intuitively that stopping the drugs, putting a line under the cancer treatment and getting on with our lives again was what we wanted to do. We were very fortunate that I quickly became pregnant. I had a trouble free pregnancy and then a very healthy baby, who I even managed to breastfeed (from the untreated breast) for nearly a year.

When Lucy wrote this piece, it opened up many raw emotions. As with any traumatic major life event, we may learn eventually, to adapt to a new situation. But the feelings evoked by an experience don't necessarily go away. They lie dormant and sometimes, the most unexpected things can trigger a rush of emotions that can make it seem as if the events only happened yesterday. Yet many people say that over time, cancer stops dominating their lives. It can never be completely forgotten, as routine follow-up appointments don't allow that.

Lucy's postscript illustrates the feelings that were stirred up when she wrote this piece.

I've not written very much but it took a while and I've pondered over it for even longer. I've realised that I don't in any way want to be identified by it. My husband doesn't understand that and thinks that I should put my name to it and be proud of coming through the experience, but I can't quite do that. Writing about it – thinking about it all – even now makes me realise how awful it all was and how difficult and desperate I found it at times. I'm not ready to let anyone and everyone know that! I don't really know why.

> *Looking back on it I think I went back to full time work too early, I was still in shock – denial, really – and I just wanted everything to get back to how it had been before the cancer. Going back to work restored a sense of 'normality', but I didn't give myself the chance to rest, recuperate and psychologically adjust to the shock and the trauma. I ended up getting anxious and depressed, and I'm sure it delayed my full recovery.*

Surviving cancer may bring about practical problems such as financial or employment concerns. Questions may arise about life or travel insurance, obtaining a mortgage or disclosing your medical history to a future employer. As survival becomes more common, health and other professionals are responding more positively to these questions.

There is life after cancer as these three stories confirm. Time heals, although life will never be the same as it was before diagnosis. Echoing what Patricia said, the experience of cancer will change your life forever. But that doesn't mean to say that good things can't happen, although you will need to allow time to grieve for the losses in your life.

Resources

Bristol Cancer Help Centre
Grove House, Cornwallis Grove, Clifton, Bristol BS8 4PG
Helpline: 0117 980 9505
www.bristolcancerhelp.org
Bristol Cancer Help Centre offers a holistic approach to cancer care. They run a residential therapy programme that helps people to help themselves through a range of self-help techniques and complementary therapies.

Institute for Complementary Medicine (ICM)
PO Box 194, London SE16 7QZ
Tel: 020 7237 5165
www.icmedicine.co.uk
Provides the public with information on complementary medicine and details of practitioners.

The Prince of Wales Foundation for Integrated Health
12 Chillingworth Road, London N7 8QJ
Tel: 020 7619 6140
www.fimed.org
Provides information on orthodox, complementary and alternative methods of healthcare including an information pack and finding an appropriately qualified practitioner.

The Royal Marsden Hospital
The Patient Information Service
Fulham Road, London SW3 6JJ
Tel: 020 7808 2831/2811
www.royalmarsden.org
The Royal Marsden's Patient Information Service produces a wide range of booklets
on cancer, its treatments and the practical issues of coping including the booklet After
Treatment.

You can find details of your nearest Cancer Support Centre from:
CancerBACUP
3 Bath Place, Rivington Street, London EC2A 3JR
Tel: 020 7696 9003 / Cancer Information Service: 0808 800 1234 (freephone)
www.cancerbacup.org.uk
Cancer nurses provide information and emotional support on all aspects of cancer.
They also provide information on support groups throughout the country.

Macmillan Cancer Relief
89 Albert Embankment, London SE1 7UQ
Macmillan Cancerline: 0808 808 2020 (freephone)
www.macmillan.org.uk
Provides information on support groups throughout the country including the leaflet
Help is There, *which lists over 40 cancer support and care charities in the UK*

www.wholehealthmd.com
This is an American website that provides information about various complementary
therapies. For each therapy it covers: what it is; how it works; what you can expect;
health benefits; how to choose a practitioner (although this relates to American
practice, it does give useful guidance) and cautions.

Useful reading

Eat to Beat Cancer (2003) Rosie Daniel & Jane Sen, HarperCollins.
ISBN: 0 00714 704 X.
A new book based on the nutritional approach followed by the Bristol Cancer Help
Centre.

Healing Foods (1996) Rosy Daniel, HarperCollins. ISBN: 0 722531 280 6
Written by the former medical director of the Bristol Cancer Help Centre.

Healing Foods Cookbook (2000) Jane Sen, HarperCollins. ISBN: 0 00710 816 8
A book of recipes used at the Bristol Cancer Help Centre.

8
Other problems affecting communication

We are shaped by every experience we live through. This, in turn, determines how we cope with different situations. Our beliefs and way of looking at the world are influenced by many different factors such as our families, education, employment, culture and faith, physical and emotional health, and the society we live in. If we are confronted with serious illness, all of these factors will have a bearing on how we cope and adjust to this new situation. Communicating effectively in day-to-day life can be difficult at the best of times. Communicating effectively to find the information you need to help you live with cancer may be even more of a challenge.

Additional challenges can create barriers to communication, but these can often be overcome with thoughtful insight on the part of both individual and health professional. This chapter looks at some of the issues that may create further communication difficulties, and shares ways that other people have found effective for overcoming them. If any of the following issues are important for you, it is important to let people know.

Sight difficulties

In all our relationships with the people around us we use our senses – sight, hearing, touch – to inform us. We bring together the information gathered by our senses to reach an understanding of the world we live in. For many people, this happens on a subconscious level until a difficulty is experienced that changes what previously has been taken for granted.

Sight difficulties do not merely involve written information, although we often take the availability of the written word for granted. While written information should never be seen as a substitute for face-to-face communication, it can be invaluable as back-up. When we talk with people, however, we are not just listening to the spoken word. We watch for the unspoken words that are communicated in body language – little gestures that, when combined with the words uttered, convey meaning and help us to understand. It can be much harder to guess another person's thoughts over the telephone than it may be with that person in front of you.

If you are blind or partially sighted, you will need information in a format other than standard print. This applies not only to information about your diagnosis, treatment and care. Appointment cards, letters and labelling on medication are also in written form.

Other methods of communication that can be used by people with impaired vision include:

- Braille
- Computer disk
- E-mail
- Large print
- Telephone
- Tape

The Royal National Institute for the Blind (RNIB) brings to our attention the fact that many blind and partially sighted people can read print if it is large and clear, although this may be only with great difficulty. Reading a long document can be slow and tiring. While it should be obvious that reading can be a problem, it is easy to forget that writing too can create difficulties. People who develop visual impairments later in life can often still write by hand. This may cause concern when it comes to giving consent for investigations, treatment and care. Consent can be written, oral or non-verbal and a signature on a consent form does not itself prove the consent is valid. Consent forms exist to record an individual's decision following discussions that have taken place. If you are unable to sign a consent form, this does not mean that you can't give your consent to a procedure. The RNIB suggest the use of signature guides, which show the blind person where to sign.

Larger print is essential for many blind and partially sighted people. If you can read written information in large print, tell your health professionals what size print is most suitable for you. It should be possible to enlarge some literature, making it more useful. If you are blind or partially sighted, health professionals are more likely to agree to a request for a consultation to be tape-recorded. Ask if there are any pre-recorded audio-cassettes available on your disease and treatment. People who can't see clearly may find it difficult to locate specific passages on the tape if tapes are not marked, and many elderly people find the controls on the recorder or player difficult to use.

Some blind and partially sighted people prefer particular types of information in Braille, which is a system of raised dots that can be read with the fingertips. It may be possible to request information to be produced in Braille. However, peripheral neuropathy (numbness in the fingers – a side effect of some chemotherapy drugs) causes loss or change of sensation in the fingertips. This is something you will need to be aware of if you are a Braille user.

Many blind and partially sighted people can access the Internet using a computer. Some may use the same equipment as sighted people while others may use large screens for text magnification, voice synthesizers or Braille output devices.

Don't be afraid to tell each health professional you come into contact with if you have any difficulties that could make communication harder for you. It may be that you have to remind them each time you see them, but it's worth it if you are able to feel confident that you won't miss anything important.

Hearing difficulties

Impaired hearing can add considerable anxiety to an already difficult consultation. If this is a problem for you, think about what you need to prevent it from becoming a barrier to receiving the information you need. At the beginning of your session with a doctor, nurse or other health professional, tell them that you can't hear well, and get them to write things down. Remember to take a hearing aid with you to appointments if you wear one. Taking someone with you can be especially helpful to ensure that vital information is heard and understood. It may not always be possible to be accompanied or perhaps you prefer to go on your own. If you are worried that you may not hear your name called out, you may find it helpful to tell the reception staff you have difficulty hearing and tell them where you will be sitting.

As background noise can often be a problem, ask to talk with your doctor or health professional in a private room rather than a busy clinic. Tell them if you lip-read and ask them to face you when speaking. Many people with impaired hearing 'face-read' rather than consciously lip-read. In order to see the other person's face and hands as clearly as possible, it is usually a good idea to have the light behind you.

Ask what written information is available to back up what you are told, or ask for important details to be written down for you. If you use sign language such as British Sign Language or the Deaf Alphabet, ask whether there is an interpreter in that sign language who can be available during the consultation. Unfortunately, people may need to be reminded on each occasion that you have difficulty hearing. While this may feel awkward, especially when the other person appears to forget halfway through a conversation, you need to be sure that you understand what is being said to you in order to respond appropriately. The concentration needed to take in new facts can be very tiring so ask for information to be given to you in 'bite-sized chunks'. If you are on your own, you may be worried about whether you have heard everything. Doctors are often happy to talk to a family member at a later stage, when you have given your permission for them to do this.

The Internet can be an invaluable resource and there are specific sites for deaf people and most UK charities for deaf people have their own websites.

Textphones are terminals used by deaf and speech impaired people. They have a small keyboard and a display screen and allow the user to type conversations into the telephone direct to other people who have them and to receive typed responses. Minicom is a well-known make and is often used to describe any textphone. Many organisations, both statutory and voluntary, give a textphone number as well as an ordinary telephone number. You can also call someone with a voice telephone using a textphone and a hearing person with a voice telephone can call you direct on your textphone. This service is offered through BT TextDirect, a new system, which uses the Royal National Institute for the Deaf (RNID) Typetalk service. BT TextDirect automatically connects to RNID Typetalk operators who relay text-to-voice and voice-to-text calls.

Hearing and sight difficulties

Figures from the RNIB indicate that there are around 23,000 people in the UK who have a severe loss of both sight and hearing. Some deafblind people have enough hearing to use the telephone if background noise is kept to a minimum, and the caller speaks clearly and at a pace which suits the individual. If you are able to use the telephone, tell the person you are talking to that you have a hearing loss and ask them to speak clearly and slowly. Other deafblind people use textphones (or minicoms) or Typetalk.

Some deafblind people retain enough sight to be able to use systems used by deaf people, such as lip reading, British Sign Language or the Deaf Alphabet.

Language difficulties

If English is not your first language, it may be helpful to have someone with you to act as interpreter. This could be a family member or friend if appropriate. Alternatively, you can ask whether your hospital is able to provide an interpreter. Many hospitals and other organisations use telephone interpreting services and may also have access to face-to-face interpreting services. Your GP should have this information and ideally, through the referral letter, let the hospital know if you are going to need an interpreter. Interpreters providing a face-to-face service will usually need to be booked in advance. Often there are local community organisations for people who share a common culture or ethnic background and some of them may provide an interpreting and translating service. Your local Council for Voluntary Services or a similar information service such as your local council will be able to give you details about local groups. Libraries may also have information about local organisations.

Although you may understand spoken English, you may not be so familiar with written English. Ask if there is any literature in your language, or any organisations that will be able to help.

Even when English is your first language, you will probably come across unfamiliar medical terms. Ask the doctor to explain in a different way, any term or technical word that isn't clear. It is important that you understand what you are being told and no one will think you stupid for asking for a clearer explanation.

Many adults have difficulties with reading and writing. Assumptions are made that if individuals have English as their first language, they can automatically read and write. When reading requires great concentration for a well person, illness can make the written word seem like an insurmountable hurdle. Listening to information on an audiotape or watching a video can be far less tiring. Ask if the information you want comes in any other format than the written word. Again, ask health professionals if they will agree to a request for a consultation to be recorded.

Culture

Our culture influences how we communicate with other people and it is helpful not to assume that health professionals will automatically know what is culturally important to you. If, for example, as a female, you would be more comfortable with a female health professional, ask if this can be arranged.

Some of the side effects of cancer treatments, for example body changes as a result of surgery, or hair loss from chemotherapy, can have more meaning in some cultures than in others. If a particular treatment proposed for you creates a cultural difficulty, discuss this with your doctor to see if there are alternatives. When your doctor understands why you are reluctant to accept a treatment it becomes easier to discuss all the options.

Sometimes situations arise causing problems that could so easily be avoided. The following story illustrates the lack of foresight in a radiotherapy department.

I think of all the experience I have had, radiotherapy was the worst experience. And it was worse for different reasons. The doctor explained the pros and cons about the treatment, but she didn't explain what was going to happen. You can't ask questions unless you have the information, details about the treatment, possible side effects and all of those things. I spoke to some doctor who told me to come in for simulation. He said it was measuring up for radiotherapy. It didn't make any sense to me. Nobody explained all that and the other thing nobody said is don't wear white when you come in, because they 'mark' you up. I had a white bra that got black ink on it and I had to throw it away. The other thing they did, was to use black ink on my skin. Every time I lay down they kept saying they couldn't find the marks. I got really angry towards the end and I said to them well why didn't you use a different colour. I can't be the first black person they've treated so why all this about they couldn't find the markings. About the third or fourth time I went, the nurse put some white tape where the marking should be and just put a black cross on the white tape.

Dee, breast cancer

Different cultures have different attitudes to illness and especially cancer. This can have a powerful influence when deciding with which people you feel comfortable disclosing your illness. In societies where there is a taboo about cancer, this can be very isolating. Health professionals may also make assumptions about your beliefs, based on your language, skin colour or faith. Regardless of these characteristics, everyone should be treated as an individual and encouraged to talk about what aspects of their life are important to them.

If you are from an ethnic minority even more assumptions are made. For example, sometimes people can assume you to be more religious when you may in fact you may be more secular or vice versa. You may need to make this clear.

This issue became particularly relevant in the issues relating to fertility. For example, the assumption had been made that if I was from an ethnic Islamic background I could not possibly want to store an embryo if I wasn't married. They hadn't thought to ask me if I had a boyfriend or my concern on this matter. There appeared to be much greater support for married women than for single women who may also want options on how to store eggs, embryos or embryonic tissue when undergoing chemotherapy. It is important to make clear that it is not only people with partners who are concerned about the ability to have children once their treatment is over. It may be necessary therefore to bring this subject up yourself if it has not been raised adequately.

Nina, sarcoma

Self-identity and body image

All illness, but especially cancer perhaps, can affect identity and self-image. Some of the side effects of treatment can seem particularly traumatic, particularly if there were no visible signs of illness before diagnosis. Surgery may bring about a loss whether it is visible or not.

I'd gone in for a lumpectomy and now they were telling me that I'd have to have my breast off. I might as well die because if I lose my breast that's it. I remember my friend saying to me 'Well we still love you whether you have a breast or not' and saying back to her, 'It doesn't matter about you'. I just saw that all my chances of future relationships had gone out the window. I never thought about it before. I'd always been very conscious of my breasts because when I was eleven, I had a large bust compared to my classmates. I mean, the reality is they are what is valued as being attractive; they're all part of what you are as a woman and it's no point somebody telling you it doesn't matter because it does matter. So because it's the perception that I have of myself, it's an important part of me. So how can I then take away a very important part of me and say it doesn't matter.

I went to the Cancer Resource Centre at the time of my second operation for the mastectomy and reconstruction. That was very helpful because I saw somebody who'd actually had a mastectomy. She looked normal. You don't imagine you're going to look normal for want of a better word. She looked normal and if I'd seen her walking down the street I wouldn't have known anything.

> *Your breast is such an important part of who you are. All my perception about what is female is tied up in this, all the images I was fed from the time I was small. If somebody says they're going to take it away, it's so difficult to imagine not having it. The surgeon had said he could do a reconstruction and I didn't even know what that meant, basically. The nurse specialist said to me 'You can have a reconstruction and they'll just make you another breast'. I remember saying to her but it's not the same and she said, 'No it won't be the same, it will be different'. I agreed with the surgeon that he would do it all at the same time because I could not go away and come back six months later. I said if you're going to do it, do everything all at once or not at all. He agreed that he would do a reduction in the other breast because it was quite large anyway. The nurse talked to me about it, what would happen and she showed me a book of photographs of reconstructions. Before the operation the doctor drew me pictures and told me exactly what they were going to do.*

Dee, breast cancer

Surgery can challenge the image people have of themselves as our identity is bound up with how we see ourselves physically. This is often associated with a sense of loss although the following account illustrates a positive response to dealing with such a situation.

> *I was upset and I thought I'm going to go into hospital for a couple of weeks and I'm going to come out an old woman. I'm going to come out with my hair grey and with my figure completely ruined. I didn't have a fantastic figure but I've always had a good tummy. Just before the operation, I got my oldest daughter to take some photographs of me. She was fine about taking photographs of me without my clothes. My daughter had the film developed and they were enormously comforting to me – I actually showed the nurses!*

Sadie, colon cancer

For some people, loss involves more than just physical appearance. Surgery can affect function, such as manual dexterity, for example. Loss of function can often be a constant reminder of cancer treatment, however long ago that treatment was. Meeting new people for the first time may raise questions such as 'What happened to you?' While many people find their own way of responding to such questions, depending perhaps, on how others react, the situation can become depressingly familiar.

I look at my hand and regard it as deformed. Others tell me that unless I show it, holding my hand still, the loss of my little finger and fifth metacarpal [knuckle bone] is not noticeable. However, I notice it. It feels different. It is stiff permanently. A lot of muscle has been cut away. I have reduced movement. I cannot cup my hand. I drop things, as I am clumsy. I use my left hand much more as a result. Yet I am alive, without any cancer. It helped me focus on what I wanted to do, which was to get out of a deadly job and doing what I had trained for.

Mark, sarcoma

While other changes may be temporary, they can still have a profound effect on us, especially if they are visible – like hair loss caused by chemotherapy, for example. How we wear our hair is a statement of who we are and part of our individuality. It is an important aspect of our identity, the image we have of ourselves. It is often assumed that hair loss is more of an issue for women and not a major concern for men. Men may not be able to influence the natural course of balding but at least they have control over how they deal with it, such as whether or not to shave their heads. Of course, not all chemotherapy drugs cause hair loss and even those that do may not result in total loss. Other side effects of treatment, such as lymphoedema (swelling due to build up of lymphatic fluid in the tissues), can also have a powerful effect on our body image. Our appearance contributes to our confidence and how we communicate with people.

Lymphoedema can radically affect your physical appearance and the change in body image can be a problem. Many of us who have severe lymphoedema have developed the art of defensive dressing, but there are occasions when an affected part of the body has to be put on display. The main problem is not being able to explain to people why you look different. If you could they'd no doubt be very understanding, but it's not always appropriate to talk about it. That can make one feel really uncomfortable.

Karen, breast cancer

Sexuality

One area of our lives that people frequently feel uncomfortable talking about is sexuality. It is what makes us male or female and how we relate to these identities. Sexuality is complex and unique to each individual, bringing together sexual behaviour, how we feel about ourselves and relate to others. Even when we are healthy, it is a subject that largely gets ignored.

Yet it is a vital part of our being and makes us who we are. Cancer can have an impact on sexuality in many ways, through the disease itself or as a result of treatment. But it does not just affect the individual living with cancer; it can have a profound affect on all relationships, especially relationships with intimate partners.

The period surrounding diagnosis is likely to be an anxious time, surrounded by uncertainty, when support and understanding are particularly valuable. It is not easy talking about sex and it doesn't help when health professionals seem equally embarrassed to talk about it. However, it is important to understand how cancer and its treatment may affect your sexuality. You may feel that you can talk to your doctor or a member of the team looking after you, or you could ask to be referred to someone who has experience in this area. Some hospitals may have a sexual dysfunctional clinic you could be referred to. There are also a number of organisations that you could contact for information and advice on personal and sexual relationships (see *Resources*).

Not everyone of course, is necessarily in a relationship. The thought of starting a new relationship may seem very daunting and not made any easier if there are no visible signs of bodily changes. There are no clear-cut answers as to what you may wish to tell a new partner or at what stage of the relationship. You may find it helpful to talk things through with a counsellor. Another barrier to communication can be sexual orientation and gay men and lesbians may not wish to reveal this aspect of their sexuality to the health professionals with whom they come into contact. Sex is still very important to many gay relationships and again, it may be helpful to talk through any concerns with an understanding counsellor.

Physical changes brought about through surgery can have an effect on sexuality. This may be through external changes to the body, such removal of a breast, or through removal of or damage to the sexual organs. Radiotherapy to the pelvic organs may also affect sexual function. Some of the side effects of chemotherapy, such as nausea and vomiting, hair loss, and weight changes can affect how individuals view their body and make them feel less attractive. With any of these treatments, coping with tiredness during recovery may lessen sexual desire. What is important is what your sexuality means to you and your partner and how you communicate with each other. Any problems you experience may not necessarily be permanent and seeking help could outweigh any initial embarrassment felt by talking about them.

In this next account, Melanie summarises what her cancer experience meant to her and how she coped with the impact it had on her sexuality.

At 42 years, I was the mother of two lively sons, aged 7 and 8, and the wife of a doctor. Until motherhood, I had been a Senior Ward Sister at our local hospital.

I enjoyed a happy marriage and all the challenges that motherhood brought when I first experienced the vague, episodic symptoms that were to turn my life, and that of my family, into a nightmare lasting four years. Ten years on, I continue to view my life as a very fortunate but wiser survivor.

I had spent my entire nursing career in cancer hospitals here and abroad. None of these experiences prepared us for the diagnosis of a rare but potentially fatal tumour. From a state of shock, we moved to questions about treatment and cure. We then learnt the true meaning of uncertainty and 'treatment options' that included major surgery and chemotherapy.

The operation proved hazardous and required four days management in intensive care followed by three weeks on the ward. Progress was slow and painful but by the Christmas I never thought I would see, I felt better than I had for at least two years.

This state of well being lasted six months before symptoms returned and further tests led to more major surgery. This time the recovery lasted nearly a year before the saga repeated itself followed by more surgery and chemotherapy.

I am now relatively well. I live with the reality that the treatment has left me vulnerable to other illnesses, infections or acute medical emergencies. I live with the knowledge that other small tumours may lie dormant. In fact, I live the life countless of other survivors live – grateful for the present with an occasional backward glance of fear and panic.

But survival has exerted a heavy price in my personal life in an area rarely broached by doctors or nurses – namely, sexuality and intimacy. Indeed, as a practising nurse I was equally guilty of failure in communication with patients whose personal and private life was likely to have been disrupted or devastated by disease, treatment or depression.

I have learnt that effective communication is often the first victim of a life-threatening illness. There are barriers, conscious or unconscious. For a patient, the mind is clearly focused on mortality and survival whilst thought processes become disrupted by fear, anxiety, medication or the disease process; coping mechanisms are often directed at protecting a partner and children. The patient's inner world is often a lonely one. For partners and family, similar pressures exist; the fear of loss, the need to support, coping with anxiety and fear. Their inner world can be equally lonely. The level of communication between patient and partner is not solely dictated by the strength of their relationship. Rather, it is influenced by many psychological factors only discovered under stress, and there truly is no way anyone can predict in advance how they will cope and share a threat to their own or their partner's mortality.

The four years of illness had a major impact on communication and in particular our intimate, physical relationship. At first, we find reasons for ourselves – anxiety, fear, medication, changes in body image, ill health. But finding 'reasons' does not address the difficulties that arise when the needs of a loving couple are seemingly at opposite ends of the spectrum. Sexual fulfilment whether it be cuddling, kissing or intercourse, is a rich, joyful and life-long part of many relationships; it provides comfort, relieves stress, and communicates love however much one's body image has been distorted by illness.

But what happens when partners, afraid to cause further distress, never raise the subject? When doctors and nurses discuss all aspects of care and treatment but avoid questions of the impact of a life-threatening illness on our relationships? When no one appears to notice the pain of fractured physical love or unhappiness? When we are left in ignorance about the side effects of treatment on intimacy?

What happens is that the patient and/or partner feels responsible; recrimination and anger may ensue immediately followed by feelings of guilt; frustration and loneliness often creates a wedge in a hitherto close relationship. You know 'something' has been lost but have no idea how to address it.

We had to learn the hard way. It was some years before we came to understand that the surgery had removed one of the sources of the hormones that drive the female libido – in other words, female castration. No one, at any stage of the illness, prepared us for this and one is hard pressed to find this information in any textbook.

To find a cause goes someway towards addressing the difficulties. Without guidance or advice, we have learnt to talk, to understand and have found ways to overcome what at one time appeared impossible obstacles and found our way back to the close, intimate and physical aspect of our relationship. And through this journey, we learnt that sexuality is not just about making love. It is how we see ourselves as a man and a woman. We were lucky because, with my recovery, we had time on our side. My advice to anyone, patient or partner, who finds they are facing similar problems, is to ASK for help and advice. Don't blame yourself or your partner; don't allow embarrassment or inhibitions dictate your right to happiness and fulfilment; don't wait for the professionals to ask the right questions. You have a right to as good a quality of life as possible, whatever the diagnosis.

As a nurse, I am acutely aware that the medical and nursing profession is poorly trained in understanding sexuality and sexual needs. In fact, many see sexuality in terms of appearance and grooming or in terms of sexual dysfunction and therefore fail to address the middle ground where intimacy is relevant to all patients, regardless of age, gender or orientation. As a profession we tend to wait for patients to raise the subject but most patients choose to keep private the sexual side of their partnerships. When problems occur, due to the impact of a life-threatening illness, it is difficult for patients to find the language, privacy and courage to broach the subject with their doctor or nurse. For the patient the embarrassment of trying to raise the subject is yet another stress in an already stressful situation. How much easier, if the potential problem or difficulties are raised by the professionals in a natural and normal manner! The relief that comes from such understanding is enormous and the long term benefits on the relationship immeasurable.

I now work in palliative care, looking after patients for whom conventional cancer treatment has failed. I am acutely aware that the quality of any person's life is not solely defined by cure or symptom control; it is defined by the life-enhancing relationships we have with our children, partners and friends. And for those, for whom a close physical relationship is part of a loving relationship, the loss of intimate sexuality is an enormous source of distress and pain. It is a lesson I have learnt as a patient; it is a lesson that now directs my nursing care.

It is incumbent on our profession to understand the side effects or disease process on these aspects of our patients' lives; to honestly provide information about potential side-effects; to raise the subject naturally and allow patients and partners to express their fears, doubts or confusion without inhibition.

We are more than a collection of cells, nerve fibres and hormones and our lives are defined by what goes on behind the closed doors of our homes. When we survive a life-threatening illness or trauma, our priorities and needs change long after our final outpatient appointment.

Some cancers are intrinsically linked to sexuality and prostate cancer is one. It is not easy making decisions about treatment that are likely to affect sexual functioning. Alan, who was diagnosed with early prostate cancer, shares his experience in the following account.

When the devastating diagnosis of cancer has sunk in and you realise that there's a very good chance it will be cured, you start asking questions about how it will affect your lifestyle. If there's a choice of treatment you opt for the one least likely to cause problems in the aftermath.

I had prostate cancer and was very concerned about incontinence and impotence as any man would be. It seemed that radiotherapy in my case, rather than the operation was the best bet, and so that's what I decided. Some time before the radiotherapy started, I was given hormone injections with the warning that they would decrease the libido and cause impotence. But reassurances were given that all should be well when the effect of the injections wore off, and near normality would resume.

I was in my 60s when I was diagnosed and enjoying a fairly fulfilling sex life, although I was sometimes impotent but not often enough to seek advice. I was resigned that during the injections and radiotherapy treatment I would lead a celibate life. Then as the effect of the hormone injections faded, the libido fully recovered although the impotence was about the same as before – everything seemed to be in working order generally. Also after radiotherapy I was told I would have 'retrograde emissions' which means that the sperm goes back into the bladder and not through the penis. I was rather intrigued the first time but discovered the orgasm was as good as before – if not better! Somebody said '. . . and without the mess'! Although I qualify for Viagra on the NHS and have some, I haven't yet used it. There have been many stories about side effects although the consultants at the hospital's sexual dysfunction clinic have been reassuring.

So one adjusts to the changes and they're not a great problem. You have to accept the possible inconveniences but remember you're alive and be grateful.

Resources

Breast Cancer Care
Kiln House, 210 New King's Road, London SW6 4NZ
Helpline/information: 0808 800 600 (freephone)
Textphone: 0808 800 6001 (freephone)
www.breastcare.org.uk
Provides free information and support to people affected by breast cancer, including a support group for lesbians with breast cancer.

British Association for Sexual and Relationship Therapy
PO Box 13686, London SW20 9ZH
Tel: 020 8543 2707
www.basrt.org.uk
Provides a list of sexual and relationship therapists and links to related organisations.

CancerBACUP
3 Bath Place, Rivington Street, London EC2A 3JR
Tel: 020 7696 9003 / Cancer Information Service: 0808 800 1234 (freephone)
www.cancerbacup.org.uk
Cancer nurses provide information and emotional support on all aspects of cancer. They produce a wide range of booklets and fact sheets on cancer, its treatments and the practical issues of coping including: Sexuality and Cancer.

GaysCan
7 Barons Close, Friern Barnet, London N11 3PS
Tel: 020 8368 9027
E-mail: gayscan@blothlom.dircon.co.uk
For gay men living with cancer, their partners and friends, and bereaved partners.

Relate
Herbert Gray College, Little Church Street, Rugby, Warwickshire CV21 3AP
Tel: 0845 456 1310 *or* 01788 573241
www.relate.org.uk
Provides details of local branches offering relationship counselling.

RNIB
105 Judd Street, London WC1H 9NE
Tel: 0845 766 9999 (for the price of a local call; 18001 before 0845 number for Textphone)
www.rnib.org.uk
Offers practical support and advice to anyone with a sight problem. They also provide publications, equipment, games and information about transcription and library services, magazines, Braille, Moon, large print and tapes.

RNID
19-23 Featherstone Street, London EC1Y 8SL
Tel: 0808 808 0123 (freephone) / Textphone: 0808 808 9000 (freephone)
www.rnid.org.uk
Provides a range of services for deaf and hard of hearing people. The RNID Information Line offers free confidential and impartial information on a range of subjects. These include employment, equipment, legislation, benefits and details of relevant local and national organisations that may be able to help in a different way.

9
Being heard

A good patient–doctor relationship is essential if you are going to cope with your cancer diagnosis in the best way. It is important for you to feel comfortable with your cancer specialist, and to have confidence in the recommended course of treatment and care. In a good relationship, you will understand and be able to discuss the treatment options your doctor recommends. Most people feel more in control when they are treated as individuals.

However, there may be times when you are unhappy with the decisions your doctor makes. Dissatisfaction with the patient-doctor relationship frequently results from poor communication. A doctor's personality and approach to communication will influence your relationship with him or her, and there are as many different personalities in doctors as there are doctors.

It can be very difficult to ask the right questions when you don't know what questions to ask. If you don't have all the information you need, it may be hard to understand why your doctor is suggesting a particular treatment option. Chapters 2 (*Finding your way around the cancer services*), 5 (*Making choices about treatment*) and 10 (*Seeking information, further reading and resources*) can help you with deciding what questions you may want to ask and how to find the information you need. Treatment options are more clear-cut for some types of cancer than for others. Your doctor will probably recommend treatments or a course of action based on the results of research and his or her own experience. However, doctors may not always agree on what the best treatment is, for example if there is more than one way of treating a particular problem.

Most people want their doctor to be honest and straightforward with them, even though they may be told things that they don't want to hear. Wanting your doctor to be honest doesn't necessarily mean that you want to know every detail. Understanding your own expectations of your doctor will help you to establish a good relationship with him or her. It is also important to remember that, over time, you may change your mind about how much information you want and how involved you want to be in making decisions. Many people find that illness and uncertainty make them feel vulnerable, and this makes it difficult for them to ask why their doctor has decided on a particular course of treatment. A doctor who is sensitive to you as a person, as well being concerned for you as a patient, should be able to establish a rapport with you, to earn your trust and encourage you to hope for the future.

If your relationship with your doctor is causing you anxiety, there may be ways of improving the situation before you ask for a second opinion. It may be helpful to make a special appointment with your doctor to talk through your concerns. Think about the issues involved, and how you can put them across honestly and openly without appearing to be confrontational. Tell the doctor if you are finding it difficult to ask questions or if you don't understand the information you are given. Perhaps the doctor doesn't understand what you are asking or how you really feel. It can be helpful to ask your questions in a different way, in order to get the information you want. This may have the added advantage of prompting the doctor to think of other ways of explaining information.

The science-based training that doctors undergo does not always prepare them to manage the emotional aspects of long-term illness terribly well. They too may find it hard – after all, they are only human! It is often a natural reaction to become defensive or withdraw if we feel attacked. Doctors may react in this way as a response to individuals who come across as frustrated, angry or hostile. Try not to let these emotions become barriers to communication. You may find it helpful to have a family member or friend with you, to make it easier to voice your concerns. Sometimes it may be less stressful talking to another health professional who can then discuss the situation with your doctor.

What is a second opinion?

There are several reasons for seeking a second opinion. If the doctor who discovered your cancer does not have much experience in dealing with your type of cancer, then it would be appropriate to refer you to a specialist who does. This could be within the same hospital or at another cancer centre. Not all treatment options are necessarily available in each cancer unit or centre. Examples of this could be specialist surgery or a new drug. If you are interested in considering a treatment that is not offered in your local hospital, your doctor may suggest you get a second opinion.

It is very important to ask for second and even third opinions especially with regard to the issue of the pathology of your tumour. It is surprising how many different opinions can exist on the same tumour!

I was first diagnosed with a rare embryonic soft tissue sarcoma known as a rhabdomyo sarcoma. This tumour I was told was more common in children. We chose to double-check the pathology in the US at Sloan Kettering in New York. The pathologist at Sloane Kettering felt that the tumour could have been of another type including a carcinoma.

My oncologist at the hospital (in Southern England) where I was being treated then sought a third opinion. The Chief Pathologist at a specialist cancer centre confirmed the tumour was embryonic but instead neuraectadermal: a more fitting diagnosis for my age and profile. Fortunately, the chemotherapy used to treat both forms was the same and very effective. However, I have been informed there could have been differing prognoses.

We had to pay for the copies of the histology reports, and for sending off the samples, but otherwise it was my right as a patient to ask for second and third opinions in the UK or elsewhere. By asking for a second opinion we also discovered that surgery on my tumour should not be carried out until I had had at least two doses of chemotherapy. Earlier surgery in my case would have provided my tumour time to spread. As a result, following the advice of the second specialist, the earlier planned surgery was postponed.

Nina, sarcoma

Some people seek a second opinion because they are dissatisfied with some aspect of their care. Often this is because communication has broken down, resulting in a lack of confidence in the doctor or unhappiness about the type of treatment that has been proposed. Under these circumstances, a second opinion will either reassure you that the proposed treatment is appropriate for you or suggest an alternative plan that is more acceptable to you. A second opinion can provide you with a different perspective on your options. Some doctors are more conservative and others more aggressive. There may be sound arguments for several different options; getting a second opinion can be a good way to hear some of them. Another doctor might come up with a completely different and promising option – one that your first doctor didn't think of or knew nothing about. This happens – no doctor can know everything or make the right decision all the time.

When I had spoken to a counsellor, we'd had a warm and emotional conversation, well emotional for me, I decided I wanted another opinion and this was my right. Not that I disbelieved the surgeon who told me I had a tumour but I wanted to speak to someone else, with whom I could have a reasoned conversation and ask the questions I felt constrained about asking before. I had been told that my option was surgery. It seemed that no discussion was forthcoming and I could not even raise the possibility of alternatives to surgery. Only privately did I think, well, what if there are other ways of dealing with this that the surgeon doesn't know about? Or knows of but doesn't rate? Would he be prepared to say so or even able to say so? What sort of constraints are on him?

Unfortunately, I was referred to another surgeon. I had wanted to see someone unconnected with surgery but after seeing the second surgeon, I asked to be referred to an oncologist. In this (third) conversation I was confronted by the seriousness of my position. Up to then my experience was that I had been spoken down to and abused. I felt it got in the way of understanding my condition and what it meant to me. This man spoke more as an equal. He had more medical knowledge than me but his manner was as an equal. He said the tumour I had was serious and this had a profound effect on me. Without having said anything very different from the others it seemed to go to the heart of the matter and I paid what he said a lot of attention. He said that while he might be able to treat it, surgery was the best option available to me. I left feeling I had been respected and treated as a human being, not merely another sarcoma case – nor, as mine was a rare sarcoma, as an oddity.

Mark, sarcoma

How can I get a second opinion?

While you are entitled to ask for a second opinion from a GP or specialist, you do not have an automatic right to get one. Neither can you insist on seeing a particular doctor. If your GP is unwilling to refer you for a second opinion, you may find it helpful taking someone with you for support. Alternatively you could ask to see another GP in the practice or consider changing your GP.

When it is your specialist who suggests that a second opinion would be helpful, a referral letter will be sent to the second specialist, asking for an assessment. Sometimes it is easier or feels more comfortable to ask your GP to arrange a second opinion. Your specialist will still be informed of this step as the second specialist will need medical information, such as the results of any investigations that you have already had, to help form an opinion.

There will be several providers of cancer services within each cancer network (see Chapter 2), able to treat the majority of cancers. Most people want the best treatment at a hospital convenient to them. However, some rare cancers may only be treated at regional specialist centres, which may not be local.

Getting a second opinion may not be so easy if where you live would involve you having to travel a considerable distance to visit a different treatment centre. The time spent on journeys can be tiring in itself, and you will need to think carefully about any decisions you make.

Confidence in your cancer specialist and the other members of the cancer team is an important part of getting better. While you may have good reasons for wanting to consult another specialist, good communication doesn't always happen automatically!

I had a number of questions about the diagnosis, which I desperately needed to ask the surgeon. Unfortunately, at my next appointment, he did not have the time to deal with all my questions. I asked for a second opinion to try to get some of my questions answered elsewhere. There was a lot of stress in trying to get that appointment sorted out between the hospitals. There were problems in getting the records and slides sent in time because one hospital wouldn't move without having received a letter and letters were being sent by post rather than fax or e-mail. In the end everything got there in time but I could have done without having to try to organise it myself to make sure that it all happened.

When I had my second opinion the surgeon volunteered that he would send me a copy of his letter to the first surgeon. I was seeing the first surgeon again a week later and when the letter did not arrive with me I rang the PA. She said that I could not have it because she had not been told to send me a copy. I explained that the surgeon had explicitly said a copy would be sent to me. In the end she faxed me a copy. It is fortunate that I did so because the letter never arrived with the first surgeon and when I saw him he had to rely on my faxed copy.

Ellen, breast cancer

While most doctors will not be offended if you ask for a second opinion, you shouldn't worry about upsetting anyone. It is *your* health that is in question, and it is important to be satisfied in your own mind that you are getting the best treatment available for your particular disease and circumstances.

What can I do if I am unhappy about my care?

While every hospital and health care organisation aims to provide the best care and facilities, it is unrealistic to think that there will never be any problems. These could range from concerns about cleanliness of an area, the unhelpfulness of a member of staff, the quality or availability of food, waiting times, car parking problems, through to worries about an aspect of medical care.

If you are concerned about any aspect of your care, it would be helpful to express this as soon as it becomes an issue for you. But it is not always easy to know who to talk to, and some people say that if they are feeling unwell, taking any sort of initiative can seem too much of an effort. You may be worried that saying 'the wrong thing' might have an adverse effect on your future care. If this is how you feel, it might be useful to consider the situation from the point of view of the health professional. While doctors and nurses do not always get everything right, they are usually motivated by what is best for their patients – if and when they know what this is. So, it is always helpful to know if there are areas that need to be improved. If you feel unable to approach a member of staff about a problem or are unsure of how to go about it, there is now a new service – the Patient Advice and Liaison Service (known as PALS) which can help with this.

Patient Advice and Liaison Service (PALS)

A new system of patient and public involvement is being developed through establishing a Patient Advice and Liaison Service (PALS) in every NHS trust and Primary Care Trust. Since April 2002, this new service has been providing patients, their carers and families, with on the spot help and information.

One of the aims of PALS is to sort out problems or concerns at the time they occur. Often problems can be resolved at this level, as the PALS staff will have the appropriate skills, experience and local knowledge to deal with them. It is obviously helpful if issues can be resolved before they become serious problems and PALS staff can support individuals by liaising on their behalf. PALS has been designed to enhance existing advocacy services not to replace them.

You do not have to go through PALS with a concern if you do not want to. Neither is PALS about making formal complaints or stopping you from making one. However, PALS staff will be able to inform and support you, should you wish to go through the formal complaints procedure. They will be able to give you information about the hospital's complaints policy that sets out the procedure to be followed.

How do I make a complaint?

If you have tried unsuccessfully to resolve a complaint informally, you may wish to consider making a formal complaint. The NHS complaints procedure is designed to investigate complaints about any aspect of NHS care given to you. Before you make a complaint, it is helpful to think through what you hope to achieve by making it. You will then find it easier to decide the form that your complaint will take. Examples of outcomes from complaints include an investigation and explanation, an apology, answers to questions or the action taken to prevent a similar experience happening again. Many people worry that by making a complaint, they are jeopardising their future treatment and care and relationships with health professionals. While it should not affect the medical care you are given, you may feel that there is no longer any trust in the relationship between you and your doctor if your complaint was about clinical care. In this situation, you will probably wish to have your care transferred to another doctor.

It is best to put your complaint in writing and keep a copy of this and all subsequent correspondence. It is generally easier to address your complaint to the complaints manager than to someone involved in your care. There are two stages to the NHS complaints procedure. The first stage is called 'local resolution' and the complaints manager will investigate your complaint. You should get a written acknowledgement of your complaint in two working days and then receive a full written response within 20 working days, signed by the chief executive of the NHS trust. If you are unhappy with the response to your complaint, you may wish to move onto the second stage of the NHS complaints procedure, called 'independent review'. There is no automatic right to an independent review. A 'convener', who will only look at whether your complaint has been properly investigated rather than the complaint itself, decides this.

The Patients' Association produces a booklet, *Making a complaint*, which you can find on their website (www.patients-association.com).

Independent advice

Community Health Councils (CHCs) are independent bodies that act as watchdogs for the public to ensure their voice is heard when decisions are made about health services, particularly at a local level. Their other important function is to be a source of information and advice to the public about local health services, how to access them and to help those who wanted to make a complaint. The Association of CHCs for England and Wales (ACHCEW) represents the interests of CHCs nationally, provides some training packages and a legal advice service for CHC members. However, the government intends to replace CHCs in England and introduce a new system of patient and public involvement. The timescale for this is still uncertain and, while the future is so uncertain, many CHCs have stopped providing complaints advice and support. This only applies in England, however, and Local Health Councils (Scotland) or Health and Social Services Councils (Northern Ireland) are continuing to provide advice and support to the public.

There is still a need for independent support and advice for people who wish to make a complaint against the NHS. Independent Complaints Advocacy Services (ICAS) are being developed to give people who want to complain the support they need to do so. They will be the responsibility of the new Commission for Patient and Public Involvement in Health (the Commission) through its local networks and will be fully independent and lay-led. People will be able to get support from ICAS providers through referral from PALS and through the Commission's local networks. It is envisaged that the Commission will be established at the beginning of 2003. CHCs and ACHCEW are likely, therefore, to stop around the time this book is published.

Access to your Medical Records

The Data Protection Act (1998) gives you the right to see medical records made about you, both in manual and electronic form. However, health professionals may refuse access if they believe that information in the records would affect the patient's physical or mental well being. If you would like to have access to your hospital records, you will need to make a formal request in writing. Some hospitals may have a form you can fill in instead of writing a letter. You should address the letter to the Health Records Manager at the hospital address. The hospital must make the records available within 40 days of completion of the application process. You may be charged up to £50, which includes a charge for photocopying and postage.

Confidentiality and personal medical information

You will be asked for information about yourself so that the hospital can give you proper care and treatment. Information concerning you and your illness may be shared with professionals concerned with your case. If you are receiving care from other organisations such as social services or community services as well as the NHS, they may also need to share some information about you with them.

Sometimes hospitals may need to use the information they collect for other reasons and they are required to tell you how the information you give them may be used. The main reasons are:

- Giving you health care and treatment;

- Helping the hospital to manage and plan their services to meet patient needs in the future;

- Helping staff to review the care they provide to make sure it is of the highest standard;

- Training and educating staff;

- Research approved by the Local Research Ethics Committee;

- Looking after the health of the general public;

- Managing and planning the NHS.

Hospitals should only ever use or pass on information if there is a genuine need for it. Where possible, they will remove details that can identify you. The law strictly controls the sharing of some types of sensitive personal information. Doctors will usually provide your next of kin with information about your illness, providing you have given your permission for it to be shared. They will also keep your GP informed of your progress.

User representation

The development of health care services in the past has been based on frameworks set by the government and health care professionals. This is now changing. Health care services must reflect the needs of their population. In order to do this, they need to involve people who actually use the various health services and other local people in the development of services.

User involvement in the health care sector currently has a high profile, as service providers are encouraged to seek the views of the public. The benefit of consulting with people who use health services is that this process can lead to better quality and more responsive services through listening to and understanding the needs and wishes of users.

The NHS Plan states that 'All NHS Trusts, Primary Care Groups and Primary Care Trusts will have to ask patients and carers for their views on the services they have received.' Each NHS Trust and Primary Care Trust (PCT) will need to establish a Patients' Forum with half of its members drawn from local patients groups and voluntary organisations. *The Cancer Plan* also states 'users and their carers should have choice, voice and control over what happens to them at each step in their care'.

Patients' Forums

During 2003, Patients' Forums will be established in every NHS Trust and PCT as independent statutory bodies. Membership will be made up of patients and other individuals from the local community, and one of the members will be elected on to the Trust Board. Patients' Forums are meant to provide an opportunity for people using the health services to have a direct influence on the quality of the services.

CancerVOICES Project

There are many more opportunities being made available now in the NHS for service users to make their views known to those planning and delivering cancer services. The importance of being 'patient-centred' is now a theme of government modernisation plans for the NHS. Macmillan Cancer Relief's CancerVOICES Project is a good example of a project that illustrates how people with cancer and their carers can have a real say in the provision of cancer services. Petra Griffiths, the Director of the Cancer Resource Centre (a voluntary organisation in South West London), is the London contact for the CancerVOICES Project. CancerVOICES is a national network of cancer services users including cancer self-help and support groups, health service users, carers and health professionals linked on a regional basis. Petra describes the work undertaken by this project and how people can be involved.

Since early 2002 the Department of Health, in partnership with Macmillan Cancer Relief's CancerVOICES Project, have provided some annual funds to each area through its Cancer Network. This enables a user involvement facilitator to be paid, and to refund the expenses of people with cancer and their carers, who give their services free of charge in order to do this work.

Getting involved in this way makes it possible for people to make use of their experiences of cancer services to benefit others in the present and the future. There are many ways in which this can be achieved:

- *By influencing plans for future services through being an official user representative on a Cancer Network Board or working group;*

- *By joining a review group to comment on patient information leaflets and booklets;*

- *By joining the committee of a national representative body such as bodies representing surgeons and medical and clinical oncologists;*

- *By getting involved in future agendas for cancer research, through the Consumer Liaison Group of the National Cancer Research Institute;*

- *By getting involved with the planning of a new service, such as an information and support centre in a hospital;*

- *Through acting as patient-teachers for health professionals during medical and nursing training, and during update courses.*

Information, support and training are available for people interested in acting as user representatives through the CancerVOICES team at Cancerlink/Macmillan. A national network of regional contacts is also available to provide support. Initially it may seem intimidating to be in the position of speaking on behalf of others with cancer in a formal setting with medical consultants and health service managers. However, the CancerVOICES training is a very empowering experience, and most people feel much more confident after the end of the two days.

Partnership Forums

Petra's account goes on to describe the work of regional Partnership Forums, which are being set up to cover the same area as local Cancer Networks. These bodies, which include sympathetic health professionals as well as lay people in their membership, aim to help those involved with user representation to share idea and inspiration, as well as to support each other.

Where users are acting as representatives on committees, having at least two representatives on any official body is a good way of ensuring that they don't become isolated. This also has the advantage that if one person is unavailable, users' views don't go unheard. In South West London, for example, the Chair and Vice Chair of the Partnership Forum, who are both people with cancer, are members of the Cancer Network Steering Group. They are also backed up by two other deputy chairs, who can be called on if either the Chair or Vice Chair are unavailable.

Sometimes users want to influence the direct delivery of cancer services. An example of this is a vociferous local campaign about the waiting time for radiotherapy treatments. This is a national problem needing long-term investment in machinery, staff training, and attention to staff pay levels. Nevertheless, the waiting time in one area came down from fourteen weeks to four weeks for 'non-urgent' cases, within four months of a user-led campaign being launched.

At other times very practical issues, such as the cost and availability of parking at hospitals, are the ones that would make a real difference to the quality of people's experience of cancer services.

Many people with cancer have become involved with a project known as *The Cancer Collaboratives Project*. The aim of this project is to improve users' experience of local services. It begins by asking people about their experiences, and asking them what changes they would like to see introduced. Then attempts are made to implement the changes recommended. For example, a great deal of work is being done all over the country to improve waiting times. One strategy that is being introduced to reduce these involves changing the way appointments are booked for different procedures, so that less time is wasted in waiting rooms.

Karen, whose story has been told elsewhere in this book, was a Partnership member of this project meeting with the steering group for a local network group. She has described a piece of work where Partnership representation had a positive outcome.

There has been discussion about the introduction of a patient held booklet, in which all oncology related appointments could be logged. The proposed name for this was the Patient Passport, which the Partnership representatives suggested was not appropriate in relation to oncology patients. The document is now to be called the Personal Care Plan, an altogether more sensitive and acceptable title.

The general ethos of this group seems to centre on a willingness to share information and use it for the common good. Hence, input is welcomed from all and it appears to be understood that the lay members of the group may need, from time to time, to ask slightly unorthodox questions.

Petra sums up such initiatives with the following information.

It is important that those representing others' views make sure they have a means of checking whether a particular concern is widespread or not. The CancerVOICES training covers a range of ways of seeking a breadth of views (such as surveys, questionnaires and interviews). In 2002 a report was published presenting the results of a national survey of hospital patients' experience of quality of care with one of six types of cancer – breast, colorectal, lung, ovarian, prostate or non-Hodgkins lymphoma. The report can be found on the Department of Health's website (www.doh.gov. uk/nhspatients/cancersurvey). Details of the findings for each Cancer Network and each hospital providing cancer services are also available. All the data reported in this survey is statistically significant, since any that was based on too small a sample was excluded. This makes it an excellent source of material for any user representative to use.

The CancerVOICES newsletter reports on the activities of user representatives in cancer services across the country. National conferences are another good way of spreading ideas and good practice.

Being heard is essential for effective communication. Just as it is important for you to hear the information you need to help make decisions about, and manage your treatment and care, it is equally important that your voice should also be heard. While you may not wish to be a formal user representative on a committee for instance, you can still influence the local delivery of care at many levels. This may mean having the confidence that your doctors are listening to what you have to say; whether it concerns symptoms you are experiencing or the impact of cancer on your lifestyle. At another level, you may have questions or doubts about a proposed treatment plan and want to feel reassured that your concerns are heard and responded to. Using your experience to help shape future cancer services is another way of being heard that can really make a difference. It is only through listening to the real experiences of real people that positive change can happen. Many of the health professionals you meet may have had little personal experience of being on the receiving end of health care. So being heard requires you to voice your views in such a way that they will be listened to and valued.

Resources

Cancer Resource Centre
20–22 York Road, London SW11 3QE
Tel: 020 7924 3924
www.cancer-resource-centre.org.uk
*Provides information, support and complementary therapies for people with cancer,
their families and friends, and encourages user involvement in cancer services.*

CancerVOICES at Macmillan Cancer Relief
89 Albert Embankment, London SE1 7UQ
Macmillan Cancerline: 0808 808 2020 (freephone)
www.cancerlink.org/common/voices/intro.html
*The Cancerlink team at Macmillan Cancer Relief can provide information about the
CancerVOICES project.*

Consumers in NHS Research
Support Unit, Wessex House, Upper Market Street, Eastleigh, Hampshire
SO50 9FD
Tel: 023 8065 1088
www.conres.co.uk
*Consumers in NHS Research aims to ensure that consumer involvement in Research
and Development in the NHS, Public Health and Social Care, improves the way that
research is prioritised, commissioned, undertaken and disseminated.*

Department of Health
PO Box 410, Wetherby, LS23 7LL
www.doh.gov.uk/cancer
Government documents about cancer services.

Patients' Association
PO Box 935, Harrow, Middlesex HA1 3YJ
Helpline 0845 608 4455
www.patients-association.com
*Offers a number of booklets and publications which can help individuals to make the
right decision about their healthcare and that of their family. These are available free
for download as PDF files (Adobe Acrobat required).*

Patient Advice and Liaison Services (PALS)
*Information about local PALS should be available in hospitals, GP surgeries, libraries
and community centres.*

10
Seeking information,
further reading and resources

This chapter takes you through some of the main areas covered in this book and aims to give you a springboard from which to access the information you want and need. What a book of this size can't do is to include masses of information – we can simply give pointers to the appropriate places to find it. To make this chapter easier to read, only the websites are listed. Full details of organisations mentioned here and throughout the book arc available in Appendix 1.

Information can help you to understand the challenges that a cancer diagnosis brings and enable you to feel more in control of your life. It can help you cope with both the practical aspects of the illness and its treatments, and manage any fears and anxieties you may feel. The right information can give you ideas about how to help yourself in the management of the illness.

Your reaction to your illness will be affected by your understanding of cancer, whether from family and friends or from newspapers, television, magazines or books. Often people's understanding needs updating and it is important to remember that *your* experience will be unique to you.

In recent years there has been a growth in information for people affected by cancer. For some people, the explosion of information on the Internet has helped them tap into material that was previously unavailable to them. It has also led to a situation where the amount of information can be overwhelming, particularly at a time when the ability to take in and understand it may be affected by the disease and its treatment. It is also true that there is as much misinformation around as there is good quality information. Rather than asking 'Is there any information available?', it is now a question of asking how you can get hold of it and how can you be sure that what you find is up-to-date and reliable.

An encouraging trend over the last few years is the way in which health professionals have begun to recognise the value and importance of providing information for their patients. Listening to what patients and the public want has influenced documents such as the *NHS Information Authority and the National Cancer Strategy* (NHS Information Authority, 2000). This can be found at www.nhsia.nhs.uk/cancer/pages/relevant/full.asp. The aim of this document is to ensure that accurate and understandable information about cancer is accessible to all those who need it. The main points of the strategy are given in the box below.

Patients and the public need the following:

◆ Access to reliable information about cancer prevention, screening procedures, the availability of services, and advice

◆ Fast, reliable communications about (for example) their appointments, test results, and treatment and care

◆ Sensitive, appropriate information about their diagnosis and the 'cancer journey'

◆ Information to help those who wish to make decisions about their own treatment and care, in partnership with health professionals

---

The strategy looks at the needs of different users of cancer information. As cancer affects one in three of the population, many people will wish to know if there are any steps they can take to prevent cancer or how it can be detected. Increasingly, people want to know more about the genetic aspects and individual and family cancer risk. Information needs to be available about the recognition of symptoms that could be due to cancer and how they can get a diagnosis that confirms or excludes cancer. For individuals with a cancer diagnosis, there are many more areas in which information is needed and can be helpful.

Different needs for information

Many people want to find out as much as possible about all aspects of their illness, treatment and care. However, when you are first diagnosed, it is not always easy to know what information is going to be most helpful and at what stage. So, what information could be helpful, where can you find it and who can provide you with it? There are different needs for information and the areas where it can be important. You will probably find there are three main areas.

The first area concerns how health and social services work. While you may know something of how they work, you may well want to build on your knowledge, particularly in the early stages when you are being or have just been diagnosed. This area includes information on:

- Cancer networks – what they are, what they do
- Cancer centres and units – what cancers are treated, what treatment and care are provided
- Local community health services – GPs, community health professionals
- Social services

The second area is to do with medical information about the cancer itself, including:

- Symptoms
- Investigations
- The different treatment options and likely outcome

The third area relates to the information you need to help you live with cancer. This includes:

- The physical and emotional effects of having treatment
- Coping with changes in family and social relationships
- Work
- The provision of support
- What can you do to help yourself?
- Who can help you and how?
- Practical and financial information including benefits
- Community resources
- Complementary therapies
- The future – life after cancer treatment.

Don't be surprised if you find that your need for information changes throughout your experience. This is very common. As your understanding increases, you may want to ask more specific questions.

Information about the health services

You may want to know where you can find information about local health services such as GP surgeries or dentists for a variety of reasons. Perhaps you have moved house, want to change your GP or need to register temporarily with a GP if you are staying away from home.

The NHS website www.nhs.uk is the official gateway to National Health Service organisations on the Internet. It connects you to your local NHS services and provides national information about the NHS such as what it does, how it works, and how to use it. They will have details of local GPs that you can telephone or visit to find out whether you can register with any of them.

Unfortunately, you may not always find it possible to register with the surgery of your choice. This may be because the GPs in that surgery are not accepting any new patients or the GPs decide not to accept an individual patient. You don't have to give a reason for wanting to change your GP, although your new doctor may ask why you don't want to stay with your present GP. All GPs are required to publish practice leaflets outlining basic information about the practice and the service they provide. These should be available at the practice.

If you need to see a doctor while you are staying away from home, you can ask a GP to accept you as a temporary resident and be seen as an emergency patient.

Cancer services

Chapter 1 provided an overview of the current health services in England. If you have had little experience of illness up to now, it can be very bewildering getting to grips with which health professionals do what and where. Cancer services having been going through enormous change in an effort to ensure that good quality treatment and care is available to everyone, regardless of where they live. You will be able to find many useful documents on the Department of Health (DoH) website www.doh. gov.uk/cancer. Full details of how to order their publications are given on page 151.

The available documents include:

- *The Cancer Plan 2000*

- *Referral Guidelines for Suspected Cancer 2000*
  These guidelines help GPs to identify those people who are most likely to have cancer and who should be referred on to a specialist. They can also help identify people who are unlikely to have cancer and require non-urgent referral to hospital.

The DoH has published several documents that look at how cancer services should be organised in order to provide the best treatment and care.

The National Institute for Clinical Excellence (NICE) has now taken over the responsibility for updating existing guidance and developing guidance for other cancers. The guidance documents can be found through the DoH website and where appropriate, you will be forwarded onto the NICE website (www.nice.org.uk).

The documents include:

- Clinical Outcomes Group Guidance
  Breast cancer (1996) – the original guidance has been updated by NICE for the NHS in England and Wales and is called *Improving Outcomes in Breast Cancer: Update*. They have updated some of the original recommendations, added further recommendations and have also produced information for the public.
  Colorectal cancer (1997)
  Lung cancer (1998)
  Gynaecological cancer (1999)
  Upper gastrointestinal cancers (2002)
  Urological cancers (2002)

- *The NHS Prostate Cancer Programme* (2000)

- *Good practice in consent implementation guide* (2001)

- *Consent – what you have a right to expect: A guide for adults* (2001)

The Commission for Health Improvement (CHI) and the Audit Commission undertook a large study of cancer services (*NHS Cancer Care in England and Wales*, 2001). This can be found on their websites www.nhsia.nhs.uk/cancer/pages (you can also order it from The Stationery Office on 0870 600 5522).

While these documents can be really useful in helping you to understand what the standards of cancer services should be throughout the country, you will probably want to know what is available locally. Cancer services do vary in different areas and currently, there is little national information available on these variations. Cancer Networks are beginning to develop their own websites, with access to the public, which will give details of local cancer services.

The document *Towards a Cancer Information Strategy* (2000), which can also be found at www.nhsia.nhs.uk/cancer/pages, provides more details as to what information Cancer Networks should be providing. Cancer Networks should 'publish, on paper and electronically, a Local Cancer Directory for use by the public, cancer patients and carers, and health and social care professionals.' Cancer Units and Cancer Centres should also work towards providing patients with a personalised Cancer Information Pack as early as possible after diagnosis and work towards the provision of a Cancer Information Centre or equivalent service.

This Cancer Information Pack should contain details of national services such as cancer helplines and information relating to the type of cancer and treatment appropriate for each individual. The latter information will need to meet nationally agreed standards. The pack is also to include a Local Cancer Directory, general hospital information and more specific information on an individual's treatment plan.

It is encouraging that over the past few years, there has been a marked increase in the development of cancer information and support centres in Cancer Units, Cancer Centres and the community, where much of this information already exists. However, there is still a long way to go before everyone has access to good quality and timely information, and support.

Information about cancer and the treatments available

Many people want as much information as possible about their cancer, the different treatment options and their side effects. Information can help you to understand what is happening to you and prepare you for the time ahead. It can help you to cope more effectively with any potential side effects. Wanting information does not necessarily mean that you will always want to take part in making decisions about your treatment. However, having a choice about whether to take part in decisions can help you to feel more in control.

Before you can begin to make sense of information on specific treatments, you will need to have some basic understanding of the type of cancer you have. Without this, it is difficult to put the different treatment options into any context. When you are first diagnosed, your doctor will (or should) discuss the type of cancer you have and any further investigations you may need to help decide the most appropriate treatment. You may also be given some written information to back up what has been said to you. However, at some stage you may feel you want more information, especially when you've had time to reflect on what's happening and a chance to talk to family or friends.

So where do you start looking?

Start by talking to your cancer team. Information-giving can vary considerably between different hospitals. Too much information in one go can often be overwhelming, so some health professionals may prefer to give basic facts then wait until the patient asks for more. It would also be help-ful for you to find out whether there is a Cancer Information and Support Centre at your hospital or locally in the community. Cancer Information and Support Centres will have information on many different topics in various forms such as leaflets, booklets, books, audio-cassettes and videos. Increasingly, they are able to offer guided access to the Internet. Libraries are also an excellent source of information. Although it may seem that the Internet dominates when it comes to finding information, the printed book is still with us. With printed information, you don't need any expen-sive equipment to use it, it is portable and often easier to read.

If you feel you want more information than has been offered to you at the hospital, there are a number of organisations in the UK that provide information on the different cancers, their treatment and care. These range from national to local organisations. Some are primarily concerned with research but provide general information for the public, others are more concerned with supporting people with a specific type of cancer. Information may be available in written form or through a telephone helpline. Often these organisations have websites where you can down-load information. As they are changing all the time, it is not easy to pro-vide a definitive list. More important, is how you can find them and assess the quality of information they provide. You can find examples of national cancer organisations in Appendix 1.

A key feature of the telephone helplines often provided by the national cancer information charities is their independence and anonymity. Many people contact an information service regardless of what information is available to them through their own healthcare professionals. It is one way in which they feel that they have pursued all their options before making a decision.

Information about how cancer may impact on your whole life

A cancer diagnosis will affect many aspects of your life. Often people feel the need to readjust family, social and work relationships because of issues like financial strain, personal distress, a feeling of stigma and threats to their self-image, confidence and sexuality. People respond differently to the experience of cancer and can feel vulnerable if their usual ways of coping do not work as well as they have done in the past. It's important to find a way of coping that is right for you.

Cancer is an unwanted intrusion into lives. It may cause new problems or intensify existing ones. Knowing how cancer will affect other areas of your life is just as helpful as being given information about cancer and its treatment. People often find that it gives them the opportunity to re-evaluate what's important to them, and this may lead them to make changes in their life. If all your energies have been spent on your work or family, it's not always easy to start putting yourself first. However, feeling that you are taking back some control in your life will help you to deal with your cancer in a more positive way.

Coping with cancer

Most people can remember very clearly how they were given their diagnosis of cancer. The way in which people are told is just as important as the words used, as it influences their response at the time.

It is not easy to cope with cancer on your own and people often underestimate how much support they need. Some people find that sharing the diagnosis with close family and friends can generate a great deal of support. Others may find telling those close to them very hard, especially if coping with the reaction it brings adds extra stress. Neither is it easy for family and friends to know what to say or how they can best support you. As a parent with cancer, there may be additional needs for information and support for children. There may be times when you prefer to talk to a trained counsellor or share your thoughts and feelings with others who are going through the same experience. Support groups with others in a similar position can be invaluable for some people.

There are now over 600 cancer support groups and centres nationwide, and Cancerlink (now a part of Macmillan Cancer Relief) updates a national directory of these annually. Macmillan's CancerLine (Freephone 0808 808 2020) puts people in touch with the right kind of support for them. Cancerlink also provides training and backup for people running groups, good practice guidelines and supports annual conferences of Cancer Self-Help Groups, held in Manchester and Scotland. These are organised by representatives from groups and centres across the UK. A Good Practice Resource Pack for cancer self-help and support groups is available from Cancerlink.

Cancer Support and Resource centres are also included in Cancerlink's Directory (see above), and there are discussions between some of the centres and Cancerlink/Macmillan about forming an alliance of these centres, to help raise their profile on the national level.

CancerBACUP is another cancer charity that can provide you with information about local groups and many of the national organisations for specific types of cancer such as Breast Cancer Care offer support as well as information. CancerBACUP also produces leaflets on wider aspects of the cancer experience, such as sexuality, diet and how to travel safely.

While awareness is growing amongst health professionals of local patient support groups and other organisations that can offer support or practical help to people with cancer, there are sometimes gaps. Information available within hospitals may be inadequate or out-of-date. If you have a Cancer Information and Support Centre at your local cancer unit or hospital, you should be able to find details of local and national information and support services, self-help groups, and complementary therapies. You should also be able to find out about what is available at your own hospital and how you can access these resources. There may be a support group you could join or be put in touch with. If you feel you would prefer to talk to someone outside the hospital environment, ask for details of services in the wider community. The notice boards in your doctor's surgery or the oncology department are also a good place to find leaflets advertising local support centres or groups, and it is always worth asking staff whether they know of any.

Information about complementary therapies

Many people are increasingly seeing complementary therapies as an important part of coping with cancer. If you have never experienced any complementary therapy, it can be daunting to know which therapies can be used during cancer treatment and which might be better avoided.

It is important to distinguish between alternative therapies and complementary therapies. The term 'alternative' implies that it is used instead of conventional treatment whereas the term 'complementary' indicates that it is used in conjunction with conventional treatment.

You may want to find out more about the different complementary therapies available, which ones will be most helpful and how to find a suitable practitioner. Increasingly, many cancer units and centres are offering complementary therapies although the range and access to them may well be limited. Ask what is available in your hospital. Macmillan Cancer Relief published a *Directory of Complementary Therapy Services UK Cancer Care* in 2002. This reviews the knowledge base for complementary therapies and issues surrounding their use, and provides comprehensive information on complementary therapies available in NHS hospitals and the voluntary sector. You can telephone the Macmillan Cancerline on 0808 808 2020 (freephone) to request a copy or to find details of services in your area.

Some complementary therapies may well be available through your local cancer support centre, although you may be asked to make a small financial contribution. National organisations for a particular therapy will be able to give you more detailed information and lists of practitioners. Speak to other people who have used a therapy; however, remember that what worked for them will not necessarily be the best approach for you.

The Foundation for Integrated Health (www.fimed.org) is a national organisation that provides information on different complementary therapies and how to find practitioners. You can find details about them on their website.

Information about community resources

Increasingly, there is an emphasis on trying to keep people out of hospital and, where possible, cancer treatment is given on an outpatient basis. Knowing what nursing and social services are available within your local community will help you to plan round your needs. Community support is provided by a number of services including Primary Care Trusts (PCTs) and social services. PCTs provide health care through GP (family doctor) practices and community health services. Your GP will continue to keep an eye on your medical care when you are at home. If you need other community health professionals involved in your care, such as a practice nurse or district nurse, your GP will help arrange this. You may also meet allied therapists such as physiotherapists, dietitians and speech and language therapists in the community. Social services is a department of your local council and can help you to live as independently as possible at home. They can provide different levels of care, such as personal care, depending on your needs. Sometimes a care manager, who is usually a social worker, will carry out an assessment of what help you may need and then arrange an appropriate package of care. To find out what help is available, you can contact your local social services office whose contact details should be in your local telephone book. You could also contact your local PALS (Patient Advice and Liaison Service) for more information. Should you need care from both nursing and social services, usually all the professionals involved will discuss this.

Practical and financial information

Having cancer can threaten job and financial security. While some people find they can continue working with very little disruption during treatment, others find they may need to take periods of sick leave or give up work completely. Questions can then arise about sick pay, benefits entitlement and pension rights. When people are used to being the breadwinner, it can be difficult to adjust to being the one asking for help.

Some employers are very supportive towards employees with cancer; others are less so. Depending on the type of organisation you work for, there may be clear guidelines as to what your entitlements are likely to be. Occupational health departments may be a good source of support and information and they would not discuss anything you said in confidence to your employer without your permission.

It isn't only people in paid work who have financial worries. Caring for children or other dependants can raise issues if you need to go into hospital or find you are physically and emotionally drained during treatment. Childcare arrangements also carry financial implications. Information about your options can take away some of the uncertainty and worry.

Hospital social work departments provide a service for all inpatients. They are generally part of the local council social services department but they will liaise with other social services teams as needed. Some hospitals may also have a specialist welfare rights advisor who can offer advice on welfare benefits, housing and debt issues. The Department for Work and Pensions (DWP) which has replaced the former Department of Social Security is now responsible for benefits, employment, equality, pensions and child support. Their website www.dwp.gov.uk/lifeevent/benefits/ provides an A-Z of benefits and services available through the DWP. If you've never needed to think in terms of benefits before, it can seem a daunting task to find out what you may be entitled to. Many local authorities will have advice centres that provide advice and information about benefits. Alternatively you could contact your local Citizens Advice Bureau (CAB – www.citizensadvice.org.uk).These are free, independent and confidential advice-giving agencies aimed at helping with welfare benefits, housing and money problems, family and personal matters, employment, immigration and legal enquiries. Your local CAB will be able to tell you which of these services they are able to offer.

CancerSupportUK (www.cancersupportuk.nhs.uk) is a website that has been developed to provide help, support and direction for anyone living with cancer and it currently serves the London area. It includes information about the services and other organisations that are especially for people with cancer. It also includes information and details about other non-cancer local organisations that you may find helpful. While it may not cover your area, it can give you an idea of the type of organisations that you may be able to find locally.

If you already have a social worker, they will be able to advise you on who you can contact for help with benefits.

Information about the future

Life after treatment for cancer

The need for information doesn't necessarily stop once you have finished your treatment. Although this is a time to move forward with your life, there can still be uncertainty as you readjust. Many people say that all their energy went into getting through treatment and it is only when it's finished that they have questions to ask. These may be about the long-term side effects of treatment that only now seem relevant. There are several organisations that provide information and support to people living with the side effects of their illness or treatment. Details of how to contact some of them are given in the appendix or you can contact CancerBACUP (www.cancerbacup.org.uk) for more information.

While having less frequent hospital appointments will give you more time for other important areas of your life, you may miss the security and support of regular visits. It is not unusual to worry about all sorts of symptoms in the early stages of recovery from cancer and many people find that they become anxious just before their check-ups. Your family and friends also have to readjust to this new phase.

You may find that, as a result of your experience, you have the opportunity to make new and exciting life changes. For many people, it is the first time they can consider what they want for themselves and to feel that they don't always have to put others first.

Having had cancer can have a knock-on effect on your finances, such as mortgages and insurance. Knowing where to go for financial advice can be extremely helpful. As more and more people recover from cancer, this is an area that is still neglected by financial and insurance companies.

Two booklets that address life after treatment for cancer are *After treatment*, from the Royal Marsden Hospital's Patient Information Series and *What now*, from CancerBACUP.

The Internet

The Internet is a growing source of health information. It provides access to information resources that previously would have taken time to find from organisations, in libraries and bookshops, if indeed it was available at all. One reason is that it is relatively cheap to publish documents on the Internet compared to the costs of printing. Information on the Internet can reach a far wider audience. A good example of this is the Department of Health documents. However, it can often be far from easy, not to say frustrating, to find your way around the vast amount of information that is out there. How can you find information relevant to your situation and when you do, how do you know if it is reliable? If you find information about a form of treatment, for example, on the Internet that you think might be right for your situation, take it with you when you next have a hospital appointment. Your doctors will find it easier to discuss this with you when they also have the same information.

It is not possible here to provide an in-depth guide to accessing health information on the Internet. It is a rapidly changing field and new web-sites are always appearing while established ones change or cease to exist. If you don't have access to the Internet, you might like to try your local library as many offer free access to the Internet and may also offer support to get you started if this is all new to you. Cancer information and support centres often provide guided access to the Internet. Even when you are familiar with the Internet, through work or home use, it can still be bewil-dering when faced with such an array of different websites. There are many guides which can help you connect to the Internet and guide you through searching for information. One book, *The Patient's Internet Handbook*, has been specifically written for people wanting to search for health related information.

What this section can do is to highlight some of the key areas to con-sider when using the Internet to find information.

- What sort of information are you looking for?
- How can you judge a website?
- How can you assess the quality of the information?

What sort of information are you looking for?

Deciding what information you want will help make your search easier. You may want to search the Internet for different reasons, such as finding information on:

- A specific type of cancer
- Cancer treatments
- Managing the side effects of treatment
- Complementary therapies
- Living with cancer
- Support groups
- Local health services

- Personal experiences of individuals in similar situations to your own

Knowing what you are looking for will help you to make up your mind about the type of website that will best meet your needs.

How can you judge a website?

Anyone can set up a website, from large organisations to individuals including:

- Government agencies (e.g. the Department of Health)
- Hospitals and other care providers
- National charitable organisations (e.g. Macmillan Cancer Relief, CancerBACUP)
- Pharmaceutical companies
- Local cancer support groups
- Individuals (discussing their experience of cancer, what they have found helpful, how they have dealt with problems that have arisen, etc.)

With no regulation, the quality of information on the Internet can vary enormously and you need to use it carefully. Some information may be biased and consider only one treatment option, for example, and not refer to other equally viable options. You also need to remember that information comes from many different countries. That is not to say that websites outside the UK do not have any value, but some information, particularly relating to cancer treatments, may not be relevant or appropriate in the UK.

How can you assess the quality of Internet information?

As anyone can publish on the Internet, the quality of information cannot be guaranteed. Indeed, there is as much misinformation as there is sound, evidence-based information from reputable sources. While quality initiatives are still being developed, there are some basic questions you can ask to help evaluate information from the Internet.

- *Who is responsible for the website?*
  What organisation or individual has written and designed the website? This is an indication of its reliability and a website should identify the names of the organisation and contributors.

- *Are the aims of the website clear?*
  A website should state the aims of the organisation, who it is for (health professionals, the public etc.) and what it is trying to do. Is it aiming to provide you with information; to educate you; to give you links to other places; to put you in touch with other people or to sell you something?

- *Who is the author?*
  You would expect to see the author's name in a book, magazine or newspaper article, so why not a web page. Sometimes the author's name alone, if it is familiar, is enough to help with your evaluation. In addition, you would expect them to give their affiliations, and job titles and qualifications if appropriate. Does the author refer to other authoritative work?

- *Is the information biased in any way?*
  It is important to know whether there is any conflict of interest, which could happen for instance, if the website is sponsored by a pharmaceutical company. Some pharmaceutical companies make it clear that they are providing patient information that does not promote a particular product, others are not so clear. Some websites may want to influence the way you think by only giving you information that considers one side of the story. They may, for example, only tell you about one treatment option and neglect to tell you about others that are available.

- *When was the information published or updated?*
  Information should be labelled with a publication date or a last updated date. This will help you to judge whether the information is current.

- *How can the information be checked?*
  It obviously depends on the type of information you are seeking as to what kind of evidence you should be looking for. When it comes to treatment options, it is important to know whether the information is based on an individual's opinion or if it is backed up by references to research or other evidence. These references should be clearly stated, to enable you to follow them up if you wish. Research-based information is essential to guide individuals in their decisions about their treatment and care. It may be a good idea to check other sites to see if similar information is given elsewhere.

The Internet is also a useful resource to communicate with other Internet users around the world. Individuals can communicate one-to-one or join a discussion forum and communicate with many people at the same time. There are several types of discussion forums:

- **E-mail discussion lists** use e-mails to distribute messages to a group of people interested in the same subject. Depending on the discussion group, you may find that you receive a significant number of messages a week.

- **Newsgroups** also allow you to communicate with groups of people interested in the same subject. They differ, however, in that you access the messages on a remote computer (a news server), as they are not delivered to your personal e-mail address. You send your message to the server which can then be downloaded by others.

- **Chat forums** enable you to communicate with others at the same time. Usually they work by splitting your computer screen into two parts. While you are typing a message in one part, you can read what others are typing on the other part at the same time.

Many people find these services very supportive as they can communicate with others in a similar situation. It is important to remember that the information conveyed through these discussion forums may be based on personal experiences and not on hard evidence.

Other Internet resources include:

The National electronic Library for Health (NeLH)
www.nelh.nhs.uk
The National electronic Library for Health Programme is working with NHS Libraries to develop a digital library for NHS staff, patients and the public. Their aim is to provide clinicians with access to the best current know-how and knowledge to support health care related decisions. Patients, carers and the public may also use this site.

NHS Direct Online
www.nhsdirect.nhs.uk
NHS Direct Online was launched in 1999 with the aim of providing a variety of reliable health information resources. It is the online version of the NHS Direct nurse-led telephone helpline available for 24 hours a day, 365 days a year.

Rather than trying to produce its own information on different medical conditions, NHS Direct Online is currently piloting a project to work with other providers of health information, both in the NHS and the voluntary sector. Organisations wishing to become Information Partners, will need to fulfil certain criteria to ensure that their information is produced to an acceptable standard of quality. NHS Direct Online will provide direct links to the websites of their information partners.

National Health Service organisations
www.nhs.uk
This is the official gateway to National Health Service organisations on the Internet. It provides details of local NHS services such as pharmacies (chemists), GPs, dentists, opticians, hospitals and Health Authorities in England. The website also provides information about the NHS – what it does, how it works, and how to use it.

CAREdirect
www.caredirect.gov.uk
CAREdirect is a new service being developed by the Department of Health in partnership with some local councils for people aged 60 years and older and their carers and relatives. Its aim is to make it easier for older people to get information and help when they need it. CAREdirect can help you get in touch with the organisations that provide social care, health, housing and social security benefits. Currently, CAREdirect only covers part of the country (the South West) and plans are to develop the service across England over the next few years.

The service provides local and national information about health, housing, social care and support services and social security benefits.

DIPEx
www.dipex.org
DIPEx is a new Internet-based multimedia resource that provides access to the experiences of others living with cancer, using a variety of formats including video clips, audio and written accounts. DIPEx is still being developed and at the moment, covers prostate, breast, colorectal, testicular, and cervical cancers, as well as screening for these. The project eventually aims to include experiences of all the main cancers. The project has interviewed many people who have had one of these cancers and you can watch, listen to or read their interviews. The website also provides information about an illness and its available treatments and links to

support groups and other reliable sources of medical information. Following the stories of people who have been in similar situations may help others feel that they are not alone in their experience.

The DIPEx project has been funded by a number of organisations, including the Department of Health, Macmillan Cancer Relief, the Citrina Foundation, the Consumers Association and the Lord Ashdown Trust.

Final points

These are some useful questions to ask yourself in deciding what information you need:

- What information do I need to get?
- In what way will I use the information and how will it help me?
- Who can give me the different kinds of information?
- How can I get it in a way that works for me?
- What information do I need to give and to whom?
- How can I give that information in a way that is heard?

Useful reading

The Patient's Internet Handbook (2002) by Robert Kiley & Elizabeth Graham. RSM Press, London ISBN: 1 85315 498 9

Appendix 1
Organisations and publications

Government organisations

Commission for Health Improvement (CHI)
First Floor
Finsbury Tower
103–105 Bunhill Row
London EC1Y 8TG
Tel: 020 7448 9200
www.chi.nhs.uk
CHI was established to improve the quality of patient care in the NHS by focusing on the experience of those using the services.

The Department of Health (DoH)
PO Box 777
London SE1 6XH
Fax: 01623 724524
Tel: NHS Response Line on 08701 555 455
www.doh.gov.uk/cancer
The DoH has published many documents that set out these changes. One of the best ways of finding out about them is through the DoH website. You can also obtain copies through the post by writing to them. Please quote the title and reference number for each title wherever possible.

Department of Work and Pensions
Olympic House
Olympic Way
Wembley
Middlesex HA9 0DL
Helpline 0800 88 22 00
www.dwp.gov.uk
Gives advice on benefits and information on employment rights.

The National Institute for Clinical Excellence (NICE)
Midcity Place
High Holborn
London WC1V 6NA
Tel: 020 7067 5800
www.nice.org.uk
NICE provides patients, health professionals and the public with guidance on current 'best practice' in medicine (including cancer) in England and Wales. They will be publishing further site-specific cancer guidance and more details can be found on their website. NICE reviews existing treatments and assesses new treatments for cost-effectiveness as well as other benefits.

Patient organisations

These are organisations that have been set up to provide health related (though not medical) information for the public.

CERES
PO Box 1365,
London N16 0BW
www.ceres.org.uk
CERES (Consumers for Ethics in Research) is concerned with publicising the views of patients and people participating in research and to promote informed debate about research. They produce two leaflets about medical research for the public: Medical Research and You *and* Genetic Research and You. *These list the questions you may want to ask before deciding to participate in a trial. Single copies are free (please send stamped addressed envelope).*

Patients' Association
PO Box 935
Harrow
Middlesex HA1 3YJ
Helpline: 0845 608 4455
www.patients-association.com
Offers a number of booklets and publications which can help individuals to make the right decision about their healthcare and that of their family. These are available free for download as PDF files (Adobe Acrobat required).

Patient Concern
PO Box 23732
London SW5 9FY
www.patientconcern.org.uk
Patient Concern promotes choice and empowerment for all health service users. Volunteers will answer individual patient queries (but not medical enquiries) by post if you send a stamped addressed envelope. They produce a series of leaflets including: How to survive doctors; Consent – what you need to know; How to survive anaesthesia; How to survive surgery; How to make a Living Will; How to survive the complaints procedure; How to survive medicine on the net. *Please send two first class stamps for each leaflet to cover p&p.*

Complementary therapies

Bristol Cancer Help Centre
Grove House
Cornwallis Grove
Clifton
Bristol BS8 4PG.
Helpline: 0117 980 9505
www.bristolcancerhelp.org
Bristol Cancer Help Centre offers a
holistic approach to cancer care. They run
a residential therapy programme that
helps people to help themselves through a
range of self-help techniques and
complementary therapies.

Institute for Complementary Medicine
PO Box 194
London SE16 7QZ
Tel: 020 7237 5165
www.icmedicine.co.uk
Provides the public with information on
complementary medicine and details of
practitioners.

The Prince of Wales's Foundation
for Integrated Health
12 Chillingworth Road
London N7 8QJ
Tel: 020 7619 6140
www.fimed.org
Provides information on orthodox,
complementary and alternative methods
of healthcare including an information
pack and how to find an appropriately
qualified practitioner.

Community resources

CancerSupportUK
www.cancersupportuk.nhs.uk
This website has been developed to
provide help, support and direction for
anyone living with cancer and it
currently serves the London area. It
includes information about the services
and other organisations that are
especially for people with cancer. It also
includes information and details about
other non-cancer local organisations that
you may find helpful. While it may not
cover your area, it can give you an idea of
the type of organisations that you may
be able to find locally.

The National Association of Citizens
Advice Bureaux (NACAB)
Myddelton House
115–123 Pentonville Road
London N1 9LZ
Tel: 020 7833 2181
www.citizensadvice.org.uk
NACAB will be able to give you details of
your nearest Citizens' Advice Bureau.

Relate
Relate Central Office is at:
Herbert Gray College
Little Church Street
Rugby
Warwickshire CV21 3AP
Tel: 0845 45613101
or 01788 573241
Relateline (if you need to speak to
someone immediately):
01845 130 4010
www.relate.org.uk
Provides details of local branches offering
relationship counselling.

National cancer organisations

Brain Tumour Foundation
PO Box 162
New Maldon
Surrey KT3 4WH
Tel/Fax 020 8336 2020
Provides support for people with a brain tumour, their families and professionals.

Breast Cancer Care
Kiln House
210 New King's Road
London SW6 4NZ
Helpline/information:
0808 800 6000 (freephone)
Textphone: 0808 800 6001
(freephone)
www.breastcancercare.org.uk
Provides free information and support to people affected by breast cancer.

CancerBACUP
3 Bath Place
Rivington Street
London EC2A 3JR
Tel: 020 7696 9003
Cancer Information Service:
0808 800 1234 (freephone)
www.cancerbacup.org.uk
Cancer nurses provide information and emotional support on all aspects of cancer. They produce a wide range of booklets and fact sheets on cancer, its treatments and the practical issues of coping. They also provide information on support groups throughout the country.

Cancer Research UK
PO Box 123
Lincoln's Inn Fields
London WC2A 3PX
Tel: 0800 226 237
or 020 7061 8355
www.cancerhelp.org.uk
CancerHelp UK is a free information service from Cancer Research UK about cancer and cancer care for people with cancer and their families including information about different complementary therapies.

Colon Cancer Concern
9 Rickett Street
London SW6 1RU
Helpline: 08708 50 60 50
www.coloncancer.org.uk
Provides information to people affected by colon (bowel) cancer.

Leukaemia Research Fund
43 Great Ormond Street
London WC1N 3JJ
Tel: 020 7405 0101
www.lrf.org.uk
Provides information on different types of leukaemia and related blood cancers.

Lymphoma Association
PO Box 386
Aylesbury
Bucks HP20 2GA
Helpline: 0808 808 5555 (freephone)
www.lymphoma.org.uk/support
The Lymphoma Association provides emotional support and information on a range of issues to anyone with lymphatic cancer and to their families, carers and friends.

Macmillan Cancer Relief
89 Albert Embankment
London SE1 7UQ
Macmillan Cancerline:
0808 808 2020 (freephone)
www.macmillan.org.uk
Provides free information and support for
people living with cancer.

Prostate Cancer Charity
3 Angel Walk
London W6 9HX
Helpline: 0845 300 8383
www.prostate-cancer.org.uk
Provides information and support to
people affected by prostate cancer.

The Roy Castle Lung Cancer
Foundation
200 London Road
Liverpool L3 9TA
Helpline: 0800 358 7200
www.roycastle.org
Provides information and support to
people affected by lung cancer.

Royal Marsden
The Patient Information Service
Fulham Road
London SW3 6JJ
Tel: 020 7808 2831/2811
www.royalmarsden.org
The Royal Marsden's Patient Information
Service produces a wide range of booklets
on cancer, its treatments and the practical
issues of coping.

Wessex Cancer Trust
Bellis House
11 Westwood Road
Southampton SO17 1DL
Tel: 023 8067 2200
Fax: 023 8067 2266
www.wessexcancer.org
The trust provides a wide range of
information leaflets on various aspects of
cancer and how to cope with the problems
that the disease can bring.

Organisations for conditions associated with cancer

British Association for Sexual and Relationship Therapy
PO Box 13686
London SW20 9ZH
Tel: 020 8543 2707
www.basrt.org.uk
Provides a list of sexual and relationship therapists and links to related organisations.

British Colostomy Association (BCA)
15 Station Road
Reading
Berks RG1 1LG
Tel: 0800 328 4257
www.bcass.org.uk
Provides support and non-medical information to people who have or who are about to have a colostomy.

Disabled Living Foundation (DLF)
380–384 Harrow Road
London W9 2HU
Tel: 0845 130 9177
www.dlf.org.uk
Provides a national telephone helpline service to provide immediate advice and information on equipment, gadgets and where to find them, and other organisations providing related information.

GaysCan
7 Baron Close
Friern Barnet
London N11 3PS
Tel: 020 8368 9027
E-mail:
gayscan@blothlom.dircon.co.uk
Provides support for gay men living with cancer, their partners and friends, and bereaved partners.

Ileostomy and Internal Pouch Support Group
National Secretary
Peverill House
1–5 Mill Road
Ballyclare
Co. Antrim BT39 9DR
Tel: Freephone 0800 018 4724
Fax: 028 9332 4606
www.the-ia.org.uk
Provides information and support to people who have to undergo surgery which involves the removal of their colon (colectomy) and the creation of either an ileostomy or an ileo-anal pouch.

Impotence Association
PO Box 10296
London SW17 9WH
Helpline number is 020 8767 7791
www.impotence.org.uk
Provides information, advice and support to sufferers of impotence (erectile dysfunction) and their partners.

Institute of Family Therapy
24–32 Stephenson Way
London NW1 2HX
Tel: 020 7391 9150
www.instituteoffamilytherapy.org.uk
Offers counselling for families, including those in which a family member has a serious illness or where there has been a bereavement. They also offer a service for children, young people and families facing a variety of difficulties.

Let's face it
Christine Piff
14 Fallowfield
Yateley
Hants GU46 6LW
Tel: 01252 879630
www.dgc.org.uk/LetsFace.htm
A support network for children and adults who have a 'different' face.

Lymphoedema Support Network
St. Luke's Crypt
Sydney Street
London SW3 6NH
Tel: 020 7351 4480
www.lymphoedema.org
Provides information and support to people with lymphoedema.

National Association of Laryngectomee Clubs (NALC)
Ground Floor
6 Rickett Street
London SW6 1RU
Tel: 020 7381 9993
www.24dr.com/reference/contact/group/national_laryngectomee.htm
Provides information on national clubs offering information and support to laryngectomees, their families and friends.

RNIB
105 Judd Street
London WC1H 9NE
Tel: 0845 766 9999 (for the price of a local call)
Textphone: dial 18001 before 0845 number
www.rnib.org.uk
Offers practical support and advice to anyone with a sight problem. They also provide publications, equipment, games and information about transcription and library services, magazines, Braille, Moon, large print and tapes.

RNID
19–23 Featherstone Street
London EC1Y 8SL
Tel: 0808 808 0123 (freephone)
Textphone: 0808 808 9000 (freephone)
www.rnid.org.uk
Provides a range of services for deaf and hard of hearing people. The RNID Information Line offers free confidential and impartial information on a range of subjects. These include employment, equipment, legislation, benefits and details of relevant local and national organisations that may be able to help in a different way.

Urostomy Association
Hazel Pixley
National Secretary
Central Office
18 Foxglove Avenue
Uttoxeter,
Staffs ST14 8UN
Tel: 0870 770 7931
www.uagbi.org
Provides information and support to people who have had or are about to have surgery to divert or remove their bladder.

Useful reading

There are too many books and magazines to be able to list them all here. Publications range from providing information about different cancers and their treatments to autobiographies. There is also a wealth of self-help books which can be inspirational for many people. Some of these books relate to the cancer and others are seeking to promote optimum health regardless of the readers' illness experience. Other books are really directories, sign-posting you to different organisations and resources.

After Treatment (2002) Available from The Royal Marsden Hospital's Patient Information Service (see address on page 155).

The CancerBACUP Directory of Cancer Services 2003: The Essential Cancer Information and Resource Guide for Patients, Families and Health Professionals (2002) Maurice Slevin (Editor). Class Publishing. ISBN: 1 85959 086 1

C: Because Cowards Get Cancer Too (1999) John Diamond. Vermilion. ISBN: 0 09 181665 3

Cancer at Your Fingertips (2001) Val Speechley & Maxine Rosenfield. Class Publishing. ISBN: 1 85959 036 5

Challenging Cancer (2002) 2nd ed Maurice Slevin & Nira Kfir. Class Publishing. ISBN: 1 85959 068 3

Directory of Information Materials for People with Cancer 2002/2003 (3rd edition) www.hfht.org/macmillan/index *This is a useful directory from Macmillan Cancer Relief of a selection of nationally published materials on living with cancer and treatment of different types of cancer.*

Eat to Beat Cancer (2003) Rosy Daniel & Jane Sen. HarperCollins. ISBN: 0 00714 704 X *A new book based on the nutritional approach followed by the Bristol Cancer Help Centre.*

Healing Foods (1996) Rosy Daniel. HarperCollins. ISBN: 0 72253 280 6 *Written by the former medical director of the Bristol Cancer Help Centre.*

Healing Foods Cookbook (2000) Jane Sen. HarperCollins. ISBN: 0 00710 816 8 *Recipes to accompany Rosy Daniel's Healing Foods book.*

The Journey Through Cancer: A Unique Seven-step Programme for Healing Mind and Body (2000) Jeremy Geffen. Vermilion. ISBN: 0 09 185160 2 *A book that combines a complementary approach with conventional treatment.*

Living with Cancer: Symptoms, Diagnosis and Treatments (2001) Jeffrey Tobias & Kay Eaton. Bloomsbury. ISBN: 0747554102 *Written to accompany a BBC television programme, this book looks at symptoms through to diagnosis, treatments, and possible side-effects and after-effects of cancer.*

Love, Medicine and Miracles (1999) Bernie Siegel. Rider. ISBN: 0 7126 7046 7 *A surgeon's experience of working with people with cancer, showing how people can take control of their illness.*

The Patient's Internet Handbook (2002) Robert Kiley & Elizabeth Graham. RSM Press, London. ISBN: 1 85315 498 9 *A useful resource to help you navigate the mass of on-line information.*

What Now? (2003) Available from CancerBACUP (see address on page 154).

Writing my Way Through Cancer (2003) Myra Schneider. Jessica Kingsley Publishers. ISBN: 1 84310 113 0 *A personal story of life with breast cancer, the author also looks at role of creative writing and therapy.*

i can
www.ican4u.com/
Rosemary House
Lanwades Park
Kentford
Newmarket CB8 7PW
Tel: 01638 751515
Fax: 01638 751517
i can *magazine provides information and support for everyone affected by cancer. It offers practical advice and useful explanations about cancer and its treatment, written by leading medical experts. It is published four times a year and is available to everyone free of charge. You can send your details to be added to the mailing list (subject to availability).*

Appendix 2
The Cancer Resource Centre

Set up in 1983, the Cancer Resource Centre in south London provides:

- Complementary therapies, including massage, aromatherapy and reflexology, counselling, relaxation and visualisation, therapeutic artwork, yoga, self discovery groups, spiritual healing, and creativity groups;

- Macmillan Cancer Information Service and telephone support for the local area;

- Home Visiting Service for the local area, and a *Home Visiting Service Manual* on how to set up a volunteer service for housebound people with cancer;

- Outreach Projects working with Asian and African/Caribbean people affected by cancer, and publications in Asian languages;

- A project in conjunction with CancerVOICES, encouraging user involvement in cancer services throughout London;

- Workshops and educational courses open to people from across the UK;

- Publications such as *Communication and Cancer,* and *Massage for People with Cancer.*

The Cancer Resource Centre is available to people with cancer, their families, friends and health professionals.

The Cancer Resource Centre
20–22 York Road
London SW11 3QE
Tel: 020 7924 3924
E-mail: info@cancer-resource-centre.org.uk
www.cancer-resource-centre.org.uk

Index

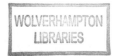

Have you found **Taking Control of Cancer** *useful and practical?*
If so, you may be interested in other books from Class Publishing.

Cancer – the 'at your fingertips' guide

THIRD EDITION £14.99

Val Speechley and Maxine Rosenfield

Straightforward, positive and practical answers to all your questions about cancer. This invaluable reference guide gives you – and people close to you – clear and practical information about cancer. Whether you have cancer yourself, or are caring for someone who does, you will find in this book the information you need to reassure yourself, and enable you to take control.

CancerBACUP Directory of Services
2003 £21.99

CancerBACUP is the leading UK organisation producing high quality cancer information for cancer patients and their families. The directory provides the only list of comprehensive treatment guidelines in the UK – and provides a unique set of documents which cover the state of the art in difficult and controversial cancer topics.

Positive Action for Health and Wellbeing – the complete programme £29.99

Dr Brian Roet

In this fascinating and original programme, Dr Brian Roet explains simply and clearly about the positive steps you can take to promote your own health and wellbeing. Using straightforward, easy and effective methods, the author shows you tried and tested steps to better health and self-esteem. Armed with this encouraging and empowering programme, you can overcome difficult problems, alleviate pain, reduce stress and tackle any fears and phobias you may have.

Challenging Cancer

SECOND EDITION £14.99

Dr Maurice Slevin and Nira Kfir

This book is not about miracles, but it is about reason, determination and concentration. This groundbreaking book gives you the information you need to feel in control of your cancer and explores the use of information, emotional support and the provision of options to help trigger changes in people's lives. It shows you how through shared experience, change and movement can emerge from chaos.

Beating Depression – the 'at your fingertips' guide £14.99

Dr Stefan Cembrowicz and Dr Dorcas Kingham

Depression is one of most common illnesses in the world – affecting up to one in four people at some time in their lives. *Beating Depression* shows sufferers and their families that they are not alone, and offers tried and tested techniques for overcoming depression.

Diabetes – the 'at your fingertips' guide

NEW! FIFTH EDITION £14.99

Professor Peter Sönksen, Dr Charles Fox and Sue Judd

This practical handbook makes it easy for you to learn more about your diabetes – and the more you know, the easier it is to manage. This updated fifth edition is an invaluable reference guide for people living with diabetes, and offers practical advice on every aspect of living with the condition, giving you the knowledge and reassurance you need to deal confidently with your diabetes.

PRIORITY ORDER FORM

Cut out or photocopy this form and send it (post free in the UK) to:

Class Publishing Priority Service
FREEPOST (PAM 6219)
Plymouth PL6 7ZZ

Tel: 01752 202 301

Fax: 01752 202 333

Please send me urgently
(tick boxes below)

Post included
price per copy (UK only)

☐ **Taking Control of Cancer**
(ISBN 1 85959 091 8)

£17.99

☐ **Cancer – 'the at your fingertips' guide**
(ISBN 1 85959 036 5)

£17.99

☐ **CancerBACUP Directory of Services 2003**
(ISBN 1 85959 086 1)

£25.99

☐ **Positive Action for Health and Wellbeing – the complete programme**
(ISBN 1 85959 041 1)

£32.99

☐ **Challenging Cancer**
(ISBN 1 85959 068 3)

£17.99

☐ **Beating Depression – 'the at your fingertips' guide**
(ISBN 1 85959 063 2)

£17.99

☐ **Diabetes – 'the at your fingertips' guide**
(ISBN 1 85959 087 X)

£17.99

TOTAL _____

Other titles in 'the at your fingertips' series £17.99 each
Contact our Priority Order Service Line on 01752 202 301

Easy ways to pay

Cheque: I enclose a cheque payable to Class Publishing for £ _____

Credit card: Please debit my

☐ Mastercard ☐ Visa ☐ Amex ☐ Switch

Number _____ Expiry date _____

Name _____

My address for delivery is _____

_____

Town _____ County _____ Postcode _____

Telephone number (*in case of query*) _____

Credit card billing address if different from above _____

_____

Town _____ County _____ Postcode _____

Class Publishing's guarantee: remember that if, for any reason, you are not satisfied with these books, we will refund all your money, without any questions asked. Prices and VAT rates may be altered for reasons beyond our control.